GW00738244

Basal Insulin Therapy in Type 2 Diabetes Mellitus

PART ONE
Insulin Glargine

Julio Rosenstock MD • David R Owens CBE, MD

Dedication

To our wives, Katty and Jennifer; only with their support, patience, understanding and love have our careers and our commitment to research and treat diabetes been possible.

Harold P. Himsworth (1905-1993) has been an inspiration to a generation of scientists and clinical researchers in type 2 diabetes. His astute keynote papers in diabetes that first recognized the twin components of deficiency of insulin or insensitivity to insulin have played a central role in current developments in our understanding of the disease. It was a great honor for me (DRO) to meet him in his later years and I would like to acknowledge his influence on my personal understanding of diabetes and on the current generation of diabetologists.

ABOUT THE AUTHORS

DR. JULIO ROSENSTOCK, MD

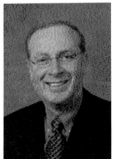

Clinical Professor of Medicine,
University of Texas Southwestern Medical Center at Dallas,
Dallas Diabetes and Endocrine Center, Dallas, Texas, USA.

Julio Rosenstock, MD, received his medical degree from the University of Costa Rica School of Medicine. He completed fellowships in endocrinology and diabetes at the Royal Postgraduate Medical School at Hammersmith Hospital in London and at the University of Texas Southwestern Medical Center in Dallas. He is board certified in internal medicine and in endocrinology and metabolism.

Dr. Rosenstock is associated with the Dallas Diabetes and Endocrine Center, an endocrine practice and clinical research facility. He is also a clinical professor of Medicine at the University of Texas Southwestern Medical Center in Dallas. His current main interest is early insulin intervention with combination strategies to reach glycemic targets in type 2 diabetes mellitus. He has more than 130 publications, including peer-reviewed papers, reviews and numerous abstracts and has also contributed to eight clinics and book chapters on various topics in the field of diabetes. He is actively involved in diabetes education as an advisory board member of CADRE. He is an editorial board member of *Practical Diabetology* and *Cardiovascular Diabetology*.

PROFESSOR DAVID R OWENS, CBE MD FRCP FIBiol

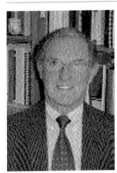

Professor and Consultant Diabetologist,
University of Wales College of Medicine,
Llandough Hospital, Penarth, UK.

Professor Owens has been involved in the field of diabetes, both treatment and research, for over 30 years and is the Director of the Diabetes Research Unit, Llandough Hospital, Cardiff, UK. For over 20 years he has been involved with a long-term study on the pathophysiology and natural history of type 2 diabetes. His continued interest in macrovascular complications of diabetes has instigated the development of the all-Wales Diabetic Retinopathy Screening Service, of which he is the Clinical Director.

His early insulin studies were published as a single author book "Human Insulin". He has a strong interest in novel insulin therapies and has written reviews on insulin analogues and on alternative routes of insulin administration. Professor Owens is a Fellow of the Royal College of Physicians and a Fellow of the Institute of Biology.

PREFACE

Our purpose in this series of books on insulin therapy is to summarize studies describing new insulin analogs in a standardized and systematic fashion and to put in perspective all the potential clinical implications and therapeutic strategies. We wished to begin this series with a review of insulin glargine (Lantus®), specifically in type 2 diabetes, for a good reason. New treatment approaches for type 2 diabetes are required and this demands new insulin therapies, in particular effective basal insulin supplementation, a requirement that has now been realized by the availability of insulin glargine. Our goal is to provide a complete overview of all the available pre-clinical and clinical evidence to date using this long acting analog.

This book has an original design, intentionally conceived and written as a structured and easily accessible guide for physicians interested in insulin therapy and its application in the context of contemporary treatment approaches in type 2 diabetes. We wished to be as extensive as possible in our search for information on insulin glargine and have included studies not only published in peer-reviewed journals, but also an exhaustive assessment of studies that have been presented and or published as abstracts at large international diabetes congresses, in particular the ADA, EASD and the IDF. This approach ensures that all studies are captured in a single structured overview, which we believe is an important contribution, as often certain abstracts and sub-analyses with preliminary or limited data, which may contain the basis for future better designed studies or may be hypothesis-generating, never find their way into the peer-reviewed literature. However, we acknowledge that this approach has certain intellectual risks and limitations. Certain abstracts contain limited information, and in all cases, an abstract is never comparable to a full, peer-reviewed paper with respect to the quantity and quality of data available for review. To account for this, all summaries of abstracts are marked clearly, in both the contents table and in the text. We caution the reader to take note of this when interpreting the data for their own clinical practice.

Academics and clinicians alike are acutely aware of potential conflicts of interest. This book was conceived and written independently from the manufacturer of insulin glargine, Aventis Pharma. We have, however, liaised with Aventis Pharma, but only to obtain data on file and with particular focus on certain clinical studies with limited information available in abstracts. Otherwise, all the description, analyses and commentaries reflect the independent views of the authors.

In Chapter One, we review the outcome studies that have demonstrated that effective glycemic control reduces the risk of microvascular and potentially macrovascular complications. This finding has prompted a major change in the type 2 diabetes management paradigm. We review the basis for the growing consensus in treatment philosophy exploring new, intensive and structured "treat-to-target" approaches. In particular, there is now a strong view that early introduction of insulin therapy, rather than regarding insulin as a last resort once other therapies have failed, is emerging as an essential component of the new treatment paradigm.

In Chapter Two, we examine the molecular chemistry of insulin glargine, and review how the modification of the molecular structure of human insulin through recombinant DNA technology has been employed to improve the kinetic profile of insulin and create insulin glargine. This chapter includes summaries of all the key pharmacodynamic, pharmacokinetic and safety studies with insulin glargine.

In Chapter Three, summaries of all clinical studies, including those that supported the licensing of insulin glargine, are presented in a standardized format. Each summary identifies the pertinent points of the study and offers our commentary. Frequently, major clinical trials are presented more than once at different international congresses, with different abstracts focusing on particular aspects of the study, or perhaps describing a substudy or additional analysis of the study. To facilitate the reader in tracking these abstracts and publications, all are listed in full under the heading "Additional References".

The downside to achieving tight glycemic control has always been hypoglycemia. There is an inevitable compromise or 'trade-off between a therapeutic strategy employing the adequate dose of insulin to achieve glycemic control and that utilizing a dose least likely to cause hypoglycemia. As introduced in Chapter 3 and detailed in Chapter 4, the benefit of insulin glargine lies in its ability to restore and maintain glycemic control within a defined therapeutic strategy at the same time minimizing the occurrence and severity of hypoglycemia. This improvement of the benefit/risk ratio with insulin glargine compared to previously available insulin preparations is examined in depth.

We hope to convey the important contribution of basal insulin therapy in the current management of type 2 diabetes. Insulin glargine provides a new opportunity for target-driven insulin treatment, used in conjunction with oral hypoglycemic agents according to need and ultimately, with prandial insulin where appropriate.

David Owens, Cardiff, Wales, UK.
Julio Rosenstock, Dallas, Texas, USA.
August 2004

"The farther backwards you can look, the farther forward you are likely to see."

Winston Churchill (1874-1965)
British Prime Minister, orator and writer

CONTENTS

CHAPTER 3

INSULIN GLARGINE: CLINICAL EVIDENCE   *87*

OVERVIEW   *92*

PHASE I AND PHASE II STUDIES   *93*

Phase I study

CHAPTER

**USING EARLY BASAL INSULIN SUPPLEMENTATION –
THE "TREAT-TO-TARGET" PARADIGM** *191*

BASAL INSULIN IN TYPE 2 DIABETES – WHY AND WHEN?

TYPE 2 DIABETES MELLITUS: THE GLOBAL EPIDEMIC

The treatment of type 2 diabetes mellitus (T2DM) and prevention of its long-term complications have become increasingly pressing clinical challenges. An estimated 18.3 million people in the United Sates are thought to have diabetes mellitus (DM) (American Diabetes Association, 2004) and every year, approximately 800,000 American adults develop diabetes. The vast majority of cases are T2DM, which is associated with advancing age, obesity, and a sedentary lifestyle. Overall, T2DM accounts for about 90% of cases, with an estimated prevalence in developed Western countries of 6–7%; an estimated one half of persons remains undiagnosed.

Worldwide, the number of cases of DM is expected to increase exponentially, with current estimates suggesting an increase from 171 million in 2000 to 371 million sufferers by 2030 (Wild et al., 2004). The increase is expected to be greatest in developing countries such as India and China, with most new cases occurring in the 45–64 year age group (Figure 1). In contrast, recent analysis of the changing world demography of T2DM confirms that most new cases in developed countries will be in the over 65 year age group and that current methods employed may offer underestimates of the size of the problem (Green et al., 2003; Wild et al., 2004).

The increased incidence of DM in young people and the longer survival of patients at risk for diabetes-related complications signal a looming health care crisis of unprecedented scope (Callahan and Mansfield, 2000). There is a responsibility at all levels, for individuals, health care professionals, the food industry and governments to attempt to counter this dire forecast by instilling the need for a better lifestyle with improved nutrition and exercise to stem this epidemic. Given that T2DM accounts for most cases, a reevaluation of the approach taken to

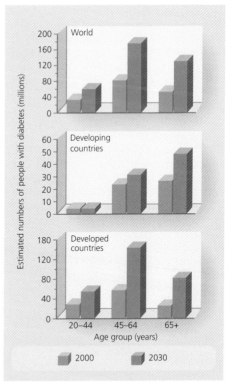

Figure 1. The global prevalence of diabetes. Estimates for 2000 & projections for 2030 by age group and country category for the developed and developing world (©2004 American Diabetes Association. From *Diabetes Care* 2004; 27:1047–1053. Modified with permission).

manage T2DM, including a reassessment of the role of insulin in reaching and sustaining glycemic targets to prevent long-term complications of T2DM, is essential (Rosenstock, 2004).

INSULIN IN TYPE 2 DIABETES – WHY?

Effective glycemic control and the prevention of long-term complications

Sustained near normoglycemia is the primary treatment goal in the prevention of diabetes-related complications. Persistent hyperglycemia in poorly controlled DM causes significant micro- and macrovascular damage resulting in long-term complications that include kidney failure, blindness, foot ulceration, amputations and heart disease, stroke, and early death. As well as the all too obvious human costs of this damage, these complications place a massive strain on the resources of health care systems.

The importance of glycemic control is highlighted by the two landmark diabetes studies, the Diabetes Control and Complications Trial (DCCT) in persons with T1DM (DCCT Research Group 1993, 1995) and the United Kingdom Prospective Diabetes Study (UKPDS) in persons with T2DM (UKPDS 33, 1998). These large, long-term studies showed important, clinically relevant reductions in the development and progression of DM-related complications, especially microvascular complications, in patients achieving target HbA_{1c} levels. The pivotal UKPDS findings in persons with T2DM are supported by two other important studies, the Kumamoto study (Ohkubo et al., 1995) and, more recently, the Steno-2 multi-factorial intervention study (Gaede et al., 2003).

The UKPDS established that the risk of retinopathy, nephropathy, and possibly neuropathy is reduced by lowering blood glucose levels with an intensive therapy approach that included insulin. The intensive therapy group achieved a median HbA_{1c} of 7.0% compared to 7.9% with conventional therapy. This improvement was associated with a significant decrease in the microvascular complication rate by 25% (p=0.0099)(UKPDS 33, 1998) (Figure 2 and Table 1).

Further findings from the UKPDS showed that the risk of DM-related complications was significantly lowered even when the HbA_{1c} was below 8.0%. Indeed, there was no evidence of any glycemic threshold for any of the microvascular complications above normal glucose levels (i.e., HbA_{1c} >6.2%)(Figure 3).

Epidemiological analysis of the UKPDS data showed a continuous association between the risk of cardiovascular (CV) complications and glycemia and showed that for each 1% decrease in HbA_{1c} (e.g. 9 to 8%), there

Variable	RR (95% CI)	p value
Any diabetes endpoint	0.88 (0.73–0.99)	0.029
Diabetes related deaths	0.90 (0.73–1.11)	0.34
All cause mortality	0.94 (0.80–1.10)	0.44
Myocardial infarction	0.84 (0.71–1.00)	0.052
Stroke	1.11 (0.81–1.51)	0.52
Microvascular	0.75 (0.60–0.93)	0.0099

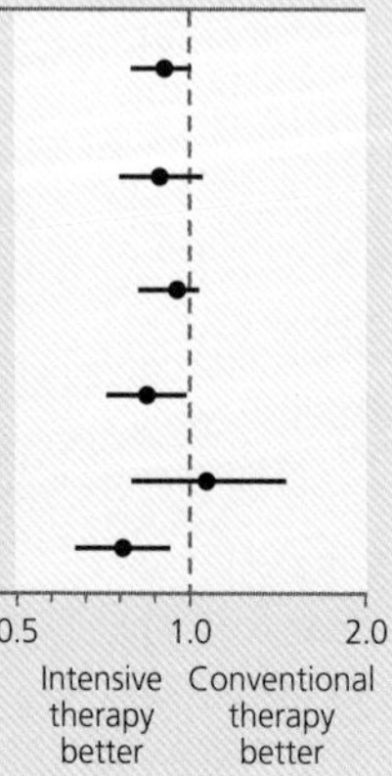

0.5   1.0   2.0

Intensive therapy better   Conventional therapy better

Figure 2. UKPDS 33 – Proportion of patients with aggregate and single endpoints by intensive and conventional treatment and relative risks (Modified from *Lancet* 1998; 352:837–853. Modified with permission from The Lancet Publishing Group).

Study name	DCCT	UKPDS	Kumamoto	Steno-2
HbA$_{1c}$	↓2%	↓0.9%	↓2%	↓0.5%
Retinopathy	↓63%	↓17–21%	↓69%	↓58%
Nephropathy	↓54%	↓24–33%	↓70%	↓61%
Autonomic neuropathy	↓60%	–	–	↓63%
Macrovascular disease	↓41%	↓16%	–	↓53%

Table 1. Reductions in HbA$_{1c}$ and corresponding reductions in microvascular and macrovascular complications described in major studies of persons with T1DM and T2DM.

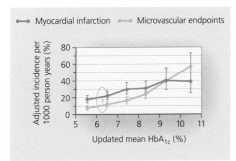

Figure 3. UKPDS 35 – Incidence rates and 95% confidence intervals by category of updated mean HbA$_{1c}$ concentration, adjusted for age, sex, and ethnic group, expressed for white men aged 50–54 years at diagnosis and with mean duration of diabetes of 10 years. The question mark indicates the uncertainty of the effect of intensive glycemic control on outcomes (Modified from *BMJ* 2000; 321:405–412, with permission from the BMJ Publishing Group).

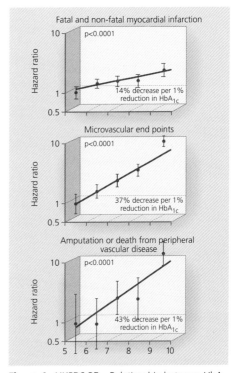

Figure 4. UKPDS 35 – Relationship between HbA$_{1c}$ concentration and risk of major adverse outcomes, for white men aged 50–54 years at diagnosis with mean duration of diabetes of 10 years, expressed as hazard ratios, with 95% confidence intervals as floating absolute risks, with a reference category (hazard ratio 1.0) based on haemoglobin A$_{1c}$ <6% with log linear scales. (Modified from *BMJ* 2000; 321:405–412, with permission from the BMJ Publishing Group).

were significant reductions in major DM-related endpoints, for example a 37% reduction in microvascular endpoints (p<0.0001), a significant 43% reduction in amputation or death from peripheral vascular disease (p<0.0001), and a significant 14% reduction in combined fatal and non-fatal myocardial infarction (p<0.0001) (Figure 4). Again, no glycemic threshold for these complications above normal glucose levels was evident.

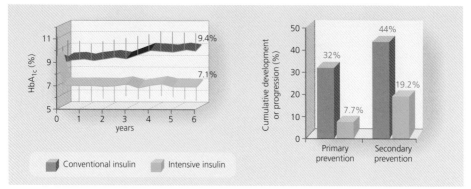

Figure 5. The Kumamoto trial. Effects of conventional vs. intensive insulin therapy and HbA$_{1c}$ reduction from 9 to 7%. The study showed a stable reduction in HbA$_{1c}$ with intensive treatment and in the cumulative incidences of change in retinopathy in the intensive treatment arm. The primary prevention cohort included patients with no retinopathy and urinary albumin secretion of <30mg/24 hours; the secondary prevention cohort included patients with simple retinopathy and urinary albumin secretion of <300mg/24 hours (data from Ohkubo et al., 1995).

Similar findings to the UKPDS have been provided by the Kumamoto study, which confirmed major reductions in retinopathy and nephropathy in persons experiencing effective restoration of glycemic control to target levels of HbA$_{1c}$ (7%) with intensive insulin treatment compared to conventional insulin treatment (Ohkubo et al., 1995) (Figure 5 and Table 1).

Outcome trials in type 2 diabetes mellitus

Despite the importance of the health problems posed by T2DM and the findings of the UKPDS, there is little definitive data on the effects of intensive control of glycemia and other cardiovascular disease (CVD) risk factors on CV event rates in patients with DM.

Completed outcome trials

The Steno-2 Study compared the effect of intensive, multifactorial intervention with that of conventional treatment on modifiable risk factors for CVD in patients with T2DM and microalbuminuria. Eighty patients were randomly assigned to receive conventional treatment in accordance with national guidelines and 80 patients to receive intensive treatment, which was characterized by a

stepwise implementation of behavior modification, followed by drug therapy targeting hyperglycemia, hypertension, dyslipidemia, and microalbuminuria, along with secondary prevention of CVD with aspirin. The principle findings are shown in Table 1 and Figure 6.

These findings from the Steno-2 study offer important insights into the value of a multi-targeted approach to DM management and a number of important long-term outcomes studies are ongoing and designed to provide more answers to these important health care questions.

Ongoing outcome trials

Three important ongoing studies are VADT (The Veterans Affairs Diabetes Trial (Abraira et al., 2003), the Action to Control CardioVascular Risk in Diabetes (ACCORD) study and the ORIGIN (Outcome Reduction with Initial Glargine InterventioN) trial.

VADT is a 5- to 7-year, randomized, multicenter trial following 1792 older patients with T2DM in the VA System in the United States. The study has been designed to answer these specific questions:

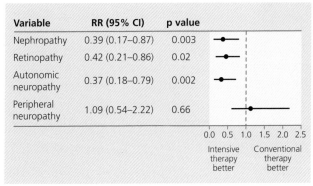

Variable	RR (95% CI)	p value
Nephropathy	0.39 (0.17–0.87)	0.003
Retinopathy	0.42 (0.21–0.86)	0.02
Autonomic neuropathy	0.37 (0.18–0.79)	0.002
Peripheral neuropathy	1.09 (0.54–2.22)	0.66

0.0 0.5 1.0 1.5 2.0 2.5

Intensive therapy better   Conventional therapy better

Figure 6. Steno-2 – The relative risk of the development or progression of nephropathy, retinopathy, and autonomic and peripheral neuropathy during the average follow-up of 7.8 years in the intensive-therapy group, as compared with the conventional-therapy group. (Reproduced from *N Engl J Med* 2003; 348:383–93. ©2003 Massachusetts Medical Society).

1. In older VA patients with established T2DM, what are the relative effects of conventional vs. intensive glycemic control on CV morbidity and mortality?
2. In this population, what is the risk-to-benefit ratio associated with intensive glycemic control?
3. Should treatment efforts be directed toward intensive glycemic control or other areas (e.g., BP management, lipid therapy, supportive care)?

The primary outcome measures are major CV events (CV death, stroke, congestive heart failure), amputation, CAD, peripheral vascular disease. Secondary outcome measures are angina, transient ischemic attack, critical limb ischemia, total mortality, retinopathy, nephropathy, neuropathy, quality of life, cognitive function, and cost-effectiveness

ACCORD is a 5-year, randomized, multicenter, double 2 x 2 factorial design trial following 10,000 patients with T2DM and high CVD risk. The study has been designed to answer these specific questions:
1. Does a strategy that targets HBA_{1C} to <6.0% reduce CVD events compared with HBA_{1C} 7.0–7.9%?
2. In the context of good glycemic control, does using a fibrate and a statin reduce CVD events compared with statin treatment alone?

3. In the context of good glycemic control, does targeting systolic BP to <120 mm Hg reduce CVD events compared with systolic BP <140 mm Hg?

The primary outcome measure is CVD morbidity and mortality. Secondary outcome measures are other CV outcomes, total mortality, microvascular outcomes, quality of life and cost-effectiveness.

ORIGIN is a 5-year, randomized, open-label, multicenter, 2 x 2 factorial design trial following 10,000 patients ≥50 years of age with at least one CVD risk factor and pre-diabetes (IFG, IGT) or early T2DM The study has been designed to answer these specific questions:
1. Does early supplementation with insulin glargine targeting fasting plasma glucose <95 mg/dL (4.7 mmol/L) reduce CV morbidity and/or mortality in high-risk patients with pre-diabetes (IFG, IGT) or early T2DM?
2. Do omega-3 fatty acid supplements reduce CV mortality in patients with pre-diabetes (IFG, IGT) or early T2DM?

The primary outcome measures are CV morbidity and/or mortality. Secondary outcome measures are MI, stroke, death, coronary artery bypass and/or coronary angioplasty, hospitalization for congestive heart failure, microvascular complications and new T2DM.

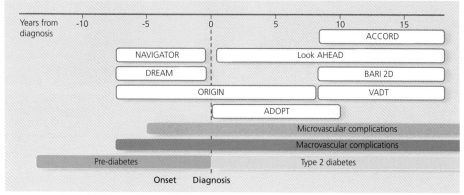

Figure 7. The natural history of T2DM progression in the context of the principal, ongoing, prospective interventional studies assessing long-term outcomes: The Navigator (Nateglinide And Valsartan in Impaired Glucose Tolerance Outcomes Research) study, The DREAM (Diabetes REduction Assessment with ramipril and rosiglitazone Medication) study, ADOPT (A Diabetes Outcome Progression Trial), ORIGIN Trial (Outcome Reduction with Initial Glargine InterventioN), the Action to Control CardiOvascular Risk in Diabetes (ACCORD) study, the Action for HEAlth in Diabetes (Look AHEAD) study, BARI 2D (Bypass Angioplasty Revascularization Investigation – 2 Diabetes) and VADT (The Veterans Affairs Diabetes Trial).

EDITORS COMMENTARY

The evidence for improved glycemic control reducing and halting the progression of DM-related microvascular complications is overwhelming. Future trials hopefully will confirm that the same is true for reducing CVD in T2DM. What is clear is that insulin will play a major role in all those interventions if the stringent glycemic targets close to normal are to be achieved and sustained.

INSULIN IN TYPE 2 DIABETES – WHEN?

Early insulin treatment in type 2 diabetes

Insulin treatment in persons with T2DM corrects glucotoxicity and lipotoxicity, improves peripheral insulin action and, by inducing "β cell rest", enhances insulin secretion. Therefore, it can be proposed that the earlier insulin is introduced, the better the potential benefit to the patient. The view that

failure to improve glucose control early can result in long-term detrimental effects on DM-related complications, despite later restoration of glycemic control because of a "metabolic memory" or "imprinting", is gaining credence in the understanding of T1DM (DCCT/EDIC, 2003) and is valuable to consider in the context of T2DM.

β cell dysfunction: a key defect in type 2 diabetes

The principal abnormalities in T2DM are impaired peripheral insulin action, insulin secretary dysfunction and increased hepatic, endogenous glucose output. Progressive impairments of both insulin secretion, as a result of pancreatic β cell dysfunction, and of insulin action in the form of insulin resistance, directly contribute to worsening glucose tolerance and thus the development and progression of T2DM (Figure 8). The increased hepatic glucose production and reduced peripheral glucose uptake result in a generalized elevation of blood glucose,

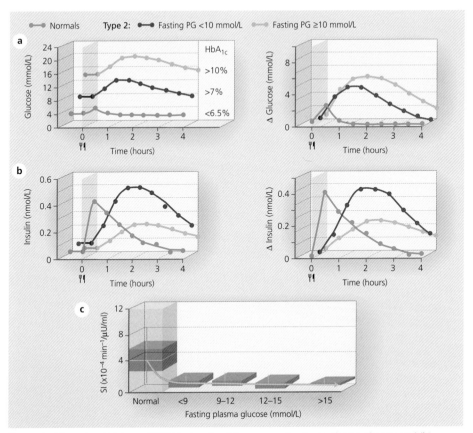

Figure 8. The natural history of T2DM, showing (**a**) a progressive rise in plasma glucose and (**b**) concomitant altered β function and impaired insulin action with (**c**) falling insulin sensitivity. In populations at high risk of diabetes, insulin resistance is present at the early stages of glucose tolerance decay and results in impaired glucose uptake (data from Coates et al., 1994).

both pre-prandial and after meals. The resulting β cell toxicity caused by hyperglycemia further undermines the metabolic milieu and coupled with reduced insulin-mediated inhibition of lipolysis, which elevates the levels of free fatty acids, further compromises β cell sensitivity and function. Usually by the time DM is diagnosed, plasma glucose levels are elevated to 126 mg/dL (7.0 mmol/L) upwards.

There is strong evidence that β cell dysfunction is a fundamental underlying genetic abnormality in the pathogenesis of T2DM.

T2DM cannot develop solely as a result of insulin resistance. β cell dysfunction is an early event which can predict the progression from normal glucose tolerance (NGT) to impaired glucose tolerance (IGT) and finally to T2DM (Weyer et al., 1999), exaggerated by the presence of insulin resistance. This key contribution of β cell dysfunction was classically demonstrated by 6-year follow-up data of the UKPDS, which demonstrated an inexorable decline in β cell function (and, therefore, insulin secretion) over time in patients with T2DM (UKPDS, 1995)(Figure 9).

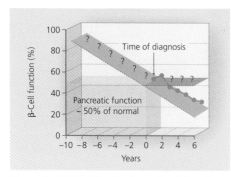

Figure 9. UKPDS 16 – Declining β-cell function over time in type 2 diabetes mellitus. The shaded area suggests the potential benefit of early introduction of insulin therapy at a time point when considerable islet function is retained (extrapolated from data from UKPDS 16, 1995).

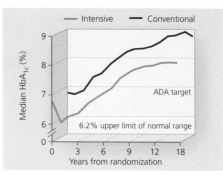

Figure 10. UKPDS 33 – Increasing HbA$_{1c}$ over time in type 2 diabetes mellitus. Even though the difference in HbA$_{1c}$ between the conventional treatment group and the intensive treatment group was about the same throughout the study, HbA$_{1c}$ progressively increased regardless of treatment. (Modifed from *Lancet.* 1998; 352:837–853. Modified with permission from The Lancet Publishing Group).

Although patients who received intensive treatment maintained significantly better glycemic control, all groups showed progressive hyperglycemia over the 6 years, with associated decrease in β cell function (Figure 10). β cell function deteriorated in the patients who were allocated to and remained on diet therapy, with a significant decrease from 1 to 6 years (53% to 26%; *P* <0.0001). Those on sulfonylurea therapy displayed an increase in β cell function during the first year of therapy (46% to 78%) that subsequently decreased significantly to 52% (*P* <0.0001) by year 6. Patients who were allocated to metformin also had an increase in β cell function in the first year that deteriorated at 6 years (66% to 38%), which was similar to that seen in the patients treated with diet alone.

A modified protocol known as the "Glucose Study 2" was introduced in the last eight UKPDS centers to determine if more aggressive glucose control could minimize hyperglycemic progression by adding insulin therapy to patients allocated to sulfonylurea therapy if maximal doses did not maintain FPG levels <108 mg/dL (6.0 mmol/L) (Wright

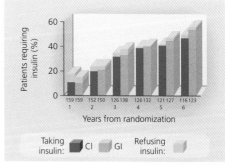

Figure 11. UKPDS57 proportions of patients (%) allocated to chlorpropamide (CI) or glipizide (GI) requiring early addition of insulin each year because FPG increased to >108 mg/dl (6.0 mmol/L) despite maximal sulfonylurea doses. Those requiring but refusing additional insulin are indicated separately. The number below each column is the number of patients per year. There were no significant differences between the chlorpropamide and glipizide groups at any time point. (©2002 American Diabetes Association. From *Diabetes Care* 2002; 25:330–336. Modified with permission).

et al., 2002). The findings are important and show that, by six years post-randomization, more than half the patients required insulin therapy in an attempt to sustain glycemic control at target levels (Figure 11).

Recent evidence has suggested that the major defect leading to a decrease in β cell mass in T2DM is increased apoptosis. In a study of pancreatic tissue from 124 autopsies, relative β cell volume, frequency of β cell apoptosis, β cell replication and the formation of new islets from exocrine ducts were measured (Butler et al., 2003). The relative rate of islet neogenesis was quantified from the percentage of exocrine duct cells that were immunoreactive for insulin.

Relative β cell volume was decreased in both obese and lean persons with T2DM, in comparison to healthy age- and weight-matched controls. In addition, subjects with pre-diabetes also exhibited decreased relative β cell volume, suggesting this is etiologically important in the development of T2DM. The study suggested that the mechanism for this was a predominance of β cell apoptosis, based on an increased apoptotic rate of β cells when normalized to β cell volume (Figure 12). This finding was independent from the rate of new islet formation. The implications for treating T2DM from this view of β cell dysfunction and increased β cell apoptosis are that strategies that avoid the increased frequency of β cell apoptosis are most rational

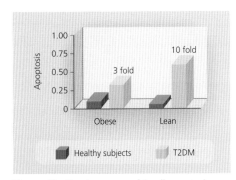

Figure 12. The frequency of β cell apoptosis normalized to relative β cell volume [(cells/islet)/(% β cell area)] based on findings from 124 autopsy samples (derived from Butler et al., 2003).

and that at least partial restoration of β cell mass may be possible if, as shown in this study, islet neogenesis remains intact.

The timing of insulin introduction – a window of opportunity

Clearly, the introduction of a therapeutic approach that supports insulin secretion and alleviates insulin resistance may have benefits that extend to the protection of β cell integrity. At the very least, early insulin therapy can offer sustained responses and improvement in glycemic control, but preliminary support for the hypothesis of insulin treatment-mediated "β cell rest" is provided by the several studies in which patients were treated with intensive insulin therapy for short periods.

In a small study in which newly diagnosed persons with T2DM received intensive insulin therapy for two weeks in an attempt to restore near-normoglycemia (Ilkova et al., 1997), most were able to sustain extended treatment-free periods of near-normoglycemia. More recently, Park and Choi (2003) showed that Korean patients with T2DM could maintain long-term normal blood glucose control without any medication after a certain period of normalization of blood glucose level by continuous subcutaneous insulin infusion (CSII) treatment. The possibility of remission was higher when the severity of glucose toxicity was lower at the initiation of therapy. These findings suggest that CSII therapy can induce remission in a significant proportion of T2DM patients.

Similarly, a recent Canadian study (Ryan et al., 2004) demonstrated that treating newly diagnosed patients with T2DM with elevated fasting glucose levels to a short (2- to 3-week) course of intensive insulin therapy can successfully lay a foundation for prolonged good glycemic control. The authors indicated that the ease with which normoglycemia was achieved may predict those patients who can later succeed in controlling glucose levels with attention to diet alone.

It is valuable to consider the importance of glycemic control in persons with T1DM. Sustained and early improvement of glycemic control through intensive treatment intervention in patients with T1DM is associated with long-term reductions in major DM-related complications (reported in the long-term follow-up of DCCT in the Epidemiology of Diabetes Intervention and Complications (EDIC) study (DCCT, 2003)). The two treatment groups in DCCT/EDIC (conventional and intensive treatment) were followed for an average eight additional years, but at levels of equivalent glycemic control during the extended time frame. The investigators concluded that the long-term, sustained improvements in outcome experienced by the intensive treatment group are explained by the early glycemic control achieved during the DCCT. This strongly supports the concept of a "metabolic memory", and that poor early glycemic control has an imprinting effect on metabolism that takes many years to overcome.

The preceding evidence offers support to the concept of insulin-mediated cessation of disease progression with early insulin intervention to preserve β cell. The current treatment debate is not about the introduction of intensive, short-term insulin, but how to introduce a low-dose insulin regimen, dictated by simple algorithms and driven by blood glucose levels to achieve near-normoglycemia with low effort, but initiated and managed in partnership with the patient. The concept of early introduction of OHAs and insulin therapy are presented in Figure 13. OHA introduction should occur as soon as the threshold target of HBA_{1c} is crossed (7%). Insulin therapy should then be presented to the patient as expected therapy, as a physiological supplementation of endogenous insulin. Once the capacity of OHAs to sustain glycemic targets is inadequate, insulin should be introduced and certainly not regarded as a treatment of last resort or, as often presented, as a threat or reflective of a patient's failure.

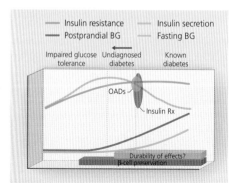

Figure 13. The natural history of type 2 diabetes, showing progressive rises in postprandial and fasting blood glucose as insulin secretion falls. The black arrow suggests the aspiration of earlier diagnosis of diabetes. The pink and red circles indicate the potential "window of opportunity" for the introduction of OHAs and insulin soon after diagnosis, before marked reduction in insulin secretory capacity, in an attempt to preserve remaining β cell capacity and positively impact on the "metabolic imprint".

EDITORS COMMENTARY

Traditionally, the requirement for insulin was seen as a 'last resort', once maximal combination oral agent therapy has failed and usually more than 10 years after the onset of T2DM. Now, an improved understanding of the underlying pathophysiology and natural history of T2DM suggests that insulin therapy should be regarded as *the* essential therapeutic tool for achieving glycemic control at the earliest stage in the natural progression of the disease. This may have further benefit and result in a favorable "metabolic imprint", helping to sustain long-term benefits by reducing progression of microvascular and macrovascular complications, which remain the ultimate objectives in the management of patients with T2DM.

References

1. Abraira C, Duckworth W, McCarren M, Emanuele N, Arca D, Reda D, Henderson W. Design of the cooperative study on glycemic control and complications in diabetes mellitus type 2: Veterans Affairs Diabetes Trial. *J Diabetes Complications* 2003; 17:314–322

2. American Diabetes Association. Diabetes Statistics at www.diabetes.org/diabetes-statistics.jsp. Accessed in June 2004.

3. Butler AE, Janson J, Bonner-Weir S, Ritzel R, Rizza RA, Butler PC. Beta-cell deficit and increased beta-cell apoptosis in humans with type 2 diabetes. *Diabetes* 2003; 52:102–110.

4. Callahan ST, Mansfield MJ. Type 2 diabetes mellitus in adolescents. *Curr Opin Pediatr.* 2000; 12:310–315.

5. Coates PA, Ollerton RL, Luzio SD, Ismail I, Owens DR. A glimpse of the 'natural history' of established type 2 (non-insulin dependent) diabetes mellitus from the spectrum of metabolic and hormonal responses to a mixed meal at the time of diagnosis. *Diabetes Res Clin Pract.* 1994; 26:177–187.

6. DCCT Research Group. The effect of intensive treatment of diabetes on the development and progression of long-term complications in insulin-dependent diabetes mellitus. The Diabetes Control and Complications Trial Research Group. *N Engl J Med* 1993; 329:977–986.

7. DCCT Research Group. The relationship of glycemic exposure (HbA$_{1c}$) to the risk of development and progression of retinopathy in the diabetes control and complications trial. *Diabetes* 1995; 44:968–983.

8. Gaede P, Vedel P, Larsen N, Jensen GV, Parving HH, Pedersen O. Multifactorial intervention and cardiovascular disease in patients with type 2 diabetes. *N Engl J Med* 2003; 348:383–93.

9. Green A, Hirsch NC, Pramming SK. The changing world demography of type 2 diabetes. *Diabetes Metab Res Rev* 2003; 19:3–7.

10. Harris MI, Flegal KM, Cowie CC, et al. Prevalence of diabetes, impaired fasting glucose, and impaired glucose tolerance in U.S. adults: the Third National Health and Nutrition Examination Survey, 1988–1994. *Diabetes Care* 1998; 21:518–524.

11. Ilkova H, Glaser B, Tunckale A et al. Induction of long-term glycemic control in newly diagnosed type 2 diabetic patients by transient intensive insulin treatment. *Diabetes Care* 1997; 20:1353–1356.

12. King H, Aubert RE, Herman WH. Global burden of diabetes, 1995-2025: prevalence, numerical estimates, and projections. *Diabetes Care* 1998 21:1414–1431.

13. Ohkubo Y, Kishikawa H, Araki E, Miyata T, Isami S, Motoyoshi S, Kojima Y, Furuyoshi N, Shichiri M. Intensive insulin therapy prevents the progression of diabetic microvascular complications in Japanese patients with non-insulin-dependent diabetes mellitus: a randomized prospective 6-year study. *Diabetes Res Clin Pract* 1995; 28:103–117.

14. Park S, Choi SB. Induction of long-term normoglycemia without medication in Korean type 2 diabetes patients after continuous subcutaneous insulin infusion therapy. *Diabetes Metab Res Rev* 2003; 19:124–130.

15. Rosenstock J. Basal Insulin Supplementation in Type 2 Diabetes: Refining the Tactics. *Am J Med* 2004; 116(3A):10S–16S.

16. Ryan EA, Imes S, Wallace C. Short-term intensive insulin therapy in newly diagnosed type 2 diabetes. *Diabetes Care* 2004; 27(5):1028–1032.

17. Stratton IM, Adler AI, Neil HA, Matthews DR, Manley SE, Cull CA, Hadden D, Turner RC, Holman RR. Association of glycaemia with macrovascular and microvascular complications of type 2 diabetes (UKPDS 35): prospective observational study. *BMJ* 2000; 321:405–412.

18. UK Prospective Diabetes Study Group. UK Prospective Diabetes Study 16: Overview of 6 years' therapy of type II diabetes: A progressive disease. *Diabetes* 1995; 44:1249–1258.

19. UK Prospective Diabetes Study (UKPDS) Group. Intensive blood-glucose control with sulphonylureas or insulin compared with conventional treatment and risk of complications in patients with type 2 diabetes (UKPDS 33). *Lancet* 1998; 352:837–853.

20. Weyer C, Bogardus C, Mott DM, Pratley RE. The natural history of insulin secretory dysfunction and insulin resistance in the pathogenesis of type 2 diabetes mellitus. *J Clin Invest* 1999; 104:787–794

21. Wild S, Roglic G, Green A, Sicree R, King H. Global prevalence of diabetes: estimates for the year 2000 and projections for 2030. *Diabetes Care* 2004; 27:1047–1053.

22. Wright A, Burden AC, Paisey RB, Cull CA, Holman RR. U.K. Prospective Diabetes Study Group. Sulfonylurea inadequacy: efficacy of addition of insulin over 6 years in patients with type 2 diabetes in the U.K. Prospective Diabetes Study (UKPDS 57). *Diabetes Care* 2002; 25:330–336.

23. Writing Team for the Diabetes Control and Complications Trial/Epidemiology of Diabetes Interventions and Complications Research Group. Sustained effect of intensive treatment of type 1 diabetes mellitus on development and progression of diabetic nephropathy: the Epidemiology of Diabetes Interventions and Complications (EDIC) study. *JAMA* 2003; 290:2159–2267.

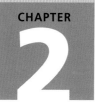

INSULIN GLARGINE CHEMISTRY AND PHARMACOLOGY

OVERVIEW

The ability to produce insulin analogs with modified pharmacokinetic properties by recombinant DNA technology has provided the opportunity to create insulin preparations that more closely mimic physiological insulin secretion patterns. Insulin glargine was designed specifically to provide the basal insulin requirement and was developed on the novel premise that the introduction of amino acid modifications that increase the isoelectric point of the native insulin molecule towards neutrality would result in precipitation of the insulin in the subcutaneous compartment and result in delayed absorption. Insulin glargine fulfilled this expectation and is characterized by delayed subcutaneous absorption and consequently prolonged action, the duration of which is almost comparable with endogenous insulin.

The successful production of novel human insulin analogs offers enormous opportunity to improve the care of persons with diabetes and correct utilization offers the best opportunity to date to mirror normal physiologic insulin secretion. However, such structural changes to the insulin protein clearly have the potential to alter kinetic and dynamic actions of the molecule and hence safety profile in a dramatic and detrimental way. Of particular interest is the insulin receptor binding properties of an analog, the binding affinity at other analogous receptors (especially IGF-1) and the associated biologic responses that such binding elicits. The studies that characterize the actions of insulin glargine with respect to these actions have been investigated in detail.

In this chapter, we describe the molecular features of insulin glargine and examine how the molecular structure directly influences its biologic effects. We present pre-clinical summaries presenting findings on receptor kinetics, signaling and mitogenicity, and on toxicology. Clinical studies describing the pharmacokinetic and pharmacodynamic characteristics of insulin glargine are reviewed in detail, including studies which have examined the influence of insulin glargine on vascular function and diabetic retinopathy. A short overview of the study and a brief description of the study design are provided in shaded boxes. In the summary, an interpretation of the relevance of these studies as a prelude to the clinical trial program for insulin glargine is presented.

MOLECULAR CHEMISTRY OF INSULIN GLARGINE

Insulin glargine (previously HOE 901) is an analog of human insulin produced by recombinant DNA technology utilizing non-pathogenic laboratory strains of *Escherichia coli* (K 12) as the production organism (McKeage and Goa, 2001). Two modifications have been made to the human insulin structure to produce the analog, insulin glargine (Figure 14)(Owens et al., 2001). Firstly, two positively charged arginine molecules have been added, which elongate the C-terminus of the β-chain. This alters the isoelectric point from pH 5·4 to pH 6·7, making the molecule, which is soluble at slightly acidic pH, less soluble at the physiologic pH of subcutaneous tissue. As insulin glargine is formulated at an acidic pH of 4.0, a second modification is needed to stabilize the insulin to prevent deamidation and dimerization via the acid-sensitive asparagine residue at position 21 in the α-chain. Neutrally charged glycine has therefore been used to replace the asparagine at position A21, to ensure good stability. When insulin glargine (pH 4) is injected into the subcutaneous space (pH 7.4), the acidic solution is neutralized, leading to precipitation. This amorphous precipitation in the subcutaneous tissue delays absorption, resulting in an extended duration of action (Figure 15).

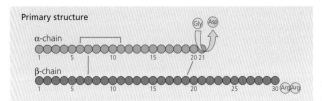

Figure 14. Insulin glargine primary structure.

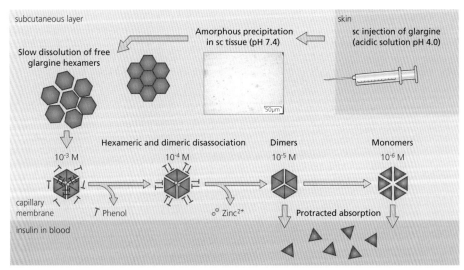

Figure 15. A representation of insulin glargine amorphous precipitation, dissociation and followed by absorption from subcutaneous tissue. The picture shows an opaque solution containing the amorphous precipitate without crystalline components under light microscopy, with no ordered structures or visible aggregates apparent. A neutralized solution of insulin glargine was prepared by injecting the drug in acidic conditions into phosphate buffered saline (pH 7.4). Image provided courtesy of Prof J Sandow, MD, PhD, Germany.

INSULIN GLARGINE FORMULATION

Chemically, insulin glargine is: A21(Gly)-B31,32 (Arg)$_2$ – human insulin. The empirical formula of insulin glargine is $C_{267} H_{404} N_{72} O_{78} S_6$. Insulin glargine has a molecular weight of 6063 daltons. Insulin glargine injection is a sterile clear solution of aqueous liquid at pH 4. Each ml of insulin glargine injection contains 100 units (3.6378 mg) of insulin glargine, 30 µg of zinc, 2.7 mg m-cresol, 20 mg of glycerol 85% and water (Lantus® Package Insert, 2002).

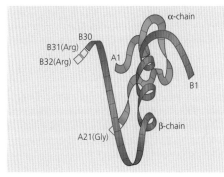

Figure 16. Insulin glargine tertiary structure.

The physicochemical properties of native human insulin have evolved to fulfill the synthesis and storage requirements for the molecule within the body. The successful storage of insulin within the granules of the pancreatic β cell is dependent on the tendency for insulin molecules to form dimeric and hexameric associations at neutral pH. Over the years, a detailed understanding of the chemistry of this process has greatly facilitated the search for replacement insulin molecules with improved pharmacokinetic properties. The association of single insulin monomers into dimers and hexamers is a complex dynamic equilibrium. The equilibrium is influenced by a number of factors, including the concentration of insulin, ionic strength, zinc and phenol content and the prevailing pH. The tertiary structure of the insulin protein (Figure 16) is based on the formation of an insulin hexamer, which is central to the formation of a globular soluble protein structure.

Insulin glargine hexamerization

The formation of an insulin hexamer is dependent on the presence of zinc ions, and, as noted, the ionic strength directly influences the equilibrium of hexamer association-dissociation (Berchtold and Hilgenfeld, 1999). The classical hexamer coordinates with six insulin molecules. The insulin molecules present in a hexamer adopt one of two conformations, the T or R state. These states reflect the spatial structure of the first eight amino acids of the β chain N-terminal, which form an extended "finger" in the T state and are α helical in the R state (Figure 17).

In the presence of small amounts of phenol or cresol molecules, which are found in commercial formulations of insulin and act as a preservative, the equilibrium is moved towards the R state. The phenolic molecules interact with the dimer-dimer interface and bind at two largely hydrophobic pockets at each dimer-dimer interface and stabilize the R state α helices. This stabilization of the R state plays a key role in stabilizing the insulin crystals because of a reduced tendency for the hexamer to dissociate. This is because the α helical shape of the B1-B8 sequence restricts zinc ion diffusion from the hexamer. Once the hexamer complexes dissociate, it is the formation of dimers and monomers, which can be absorbed through the capillary membrane, that allow biological activity (Figure 15).

Although native insulin binds six phenol molecules per hexamer (two per dimer),

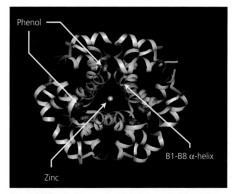

Figure 17. A diagrammatic representation of an "R" state insulin hexamer.

conformational studies with insulin glargine have shown that the glargine hexamer differs in its ability to bind phenol, and possesses the capacity to incorporate an additional (seventh) phenol molecule as a result of their novel structure (Figure 18). The extra phenol binds at the mouth of a channel created by the helical shape of the N-terminal B1-B8 sequences, and acts as a plug, reducing solvent access to the zinc ion and its ligands.

It is thought that the capacity to bind an extra phenol molecule relates to inter-hexameric association. This seems to result from distinct features of the glycine residue at position 21 in the A-chain. The 21A-Gly residue forms part of the hexamer-hexamer interface close to the seventh phenol molecule. Thus, it seems that 21A-Gly enhances the stabilization of the hexameric complex and further contributes to the protracted activity characteristic of insulin glargine. The delayed absorption

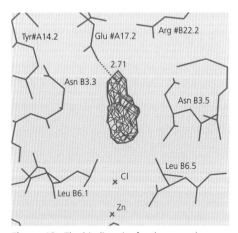

Figure 18. The binding site for the seventh phenol molecule in insulin glargine. The electron density for the phenol is displayed as heavy shading. This phenol provides an inter-hexamer link between the parent hexamer (lower half of figure) and the neighboring hexamer (upper portion of figure). Residues of the neighboring hexamer are indicated by #. The hydrogen bond between the phenolic hydroxyl group and Gly#A17.2 of the neighboring hexamer is indicated by a broken line. (Modified from *Biopolymers* 1999; 51:165–172. © 1999 Wiley Periodicals, by permission of John Wiley & Sons, Inc.).

Labels in figure: Tyr#A14.2, Glu #A17.2, Arg #B22.2, 2.71, Asn B3.3, Asn B3.5, Leu B6.5, Cl, Leu B6.1, Zn

is associated with the relatively constant insulin supply, much like that of endogenous basal insulin secretion in non-diabetic subjects in the post-absorptive state.

Insulin glargine exists as a solution at pH 4

Insulin glargine injection is an acidic solution (pH 4) and does not exist as a suspension in acidic conditions. The solution state of insulin glargine is distinct from other intermediate- and long-acting insulins. The intermediate-acting neutral protamine Hagedorn (NPH) insulin and lente insulin exist as stable protaminate suspensions formed in the presence of low concentrations of zinc. The long-acting ultralente insulin also exists as a suspension in its treatment formulation (reviewed by Barnett, 2003). The requirement to resuspend these insulin preparations before administration is a major limitation, especially for their intended use as a basal insulin required to provide peakless and stable action. There is marked inter-and intra-patient variability in the response of patients to the NPH and lente insulins, and this is particularly noted with ultralente insulin. Failure to mix adequately is common (Jehle et al., 1999), and even on vigorous mixing, reproducibility of dosing is difficult to achieve (Rosskamp and Park, 1999).

References

1. Barnett AH. A review of basal insulins. *Diabet Med* 2003:20;873–885.

2. Berchtold H, Hilgenfeld R. Binding of phenol to R6 insulin hexamers. *Biopolymers* 1999; 51:165–172.

3. Jehle PM, Micheler C, Jehle DR, Breitig D, Boehm BO. Inadequate suspension of neutral protamine Hagendorn (NPH) insulin in pens. *Lancet* 1999; 354:1604–1607.

4. McKeage K, Goa KL. Insulin glargine: a review of its therapeutic use as a long-acting agent for the management of type 1 and 2 diabetes mellitus. *Drugs* 2001; 61:1599–1624.

5. Lantus® Package Insert. Kansas City, MO. Aventis Pharmaceuticals Inc., 2002.

6. Owens DR, Zinman B, Bolli GB. Insulins today and beyond. *Lancet* 2001; 358:739–746.

7. Rosskamp RH, Park G. Long-acting insulin analogs. *Diabetes Care* 1999; 22:B109–B113.

PRE-CLINICAL PHARMACOLOGY STUDIES

Insulin and IGF-1 receptor kinetics; insulin signaling; mitogenicity

Growth promoting and metabolic activity of the human insulin analogue [GlyA21, ArgB31, ArgB32] insulin (HOE 901) in muscle cells.

Bähr M, Kolter T, Seipke G, Eckel J. *European Journal of Pharmacology*, 1997; 320:259-265.

Insulin glargine shows similar IGF-1 receptor-mediated metabolic and growth promoting activity compared to human insulin in rat muscle cell line models.

STUDY RATIONALE

Modification of the insulin molecule can lead to altered interaction with the insulin receptor and the homologous IGF-1 receptor (IGF-1R). A previous analog, Asp (B10) insulin, showed increased affinity to the insulin receptor and enhanced IGF-1R binding, which was associated with carcinogenic properties *in vivo*. Therefore, insulin glargine (HOE 901) was investigated in this context.

OBJECTIVES

To compare the growth-promoting and metabolic activities of insulin glargine and native human insulin in muscle tissue using cardiac myoblasts and rat ventricular cardiomyocytes.

STUDY DESIGN

An *in vitro* IGF-1R binding and intra-cellular signaling study undertaken in cardiac myoblasts obtained from the rat heart muscle cell line H9c2 and in adult rat ventricular cardiomyocytes.

- The IGF-1R binding and growth-promoting activity of HOE901, human insulin and Asp (B10) were investigated using the rat myoblast cell line H9c2, which expresses high levels of IGF-1R.
- IGF-1R binding was determined by incubating various concentrations of [125I]-labeled insulins with cultures of H9c2 cells

in the absence or presence of the insulins for a period of 90 minutes at 37°C. Bound radioactivity was determined by gamma counting.

- Growth-promoting activity was assessed by measuring the incorporation of [3H]-thymidine in H9c2 cells following incubation with each of the three insulins for 16 hours.
- The relative metabolic potency of the three insulin preparations was determined by measuring the uptake of [14C]-labeled 3-O-methylglucose in rat cardiomyocytes, which express high levels of the insulin-sensitive glucose transporter, GLUT4.

KEY FINDINGS

- Binding studies with IGF-1 showed high levels of IGF-1 receptor present on H9c2 cells (~7000 receptors/cell).
- Competition binding experiments using human insulin and IGF-1 indicated that the H9c2 cells did not express the insulin receptor suggesting that the effects of insulin on the cells was mediated solely by the IGF-1R.
- Competition binding experiments using [125I]-labeled IGF-1 and unlabeled human insulin, insulin glargine and Asp (B10) showed the relative strength of binding to the IGF-1 receptor to be: human insulin < insulin glargine < Asp (B10) < IGF-1 (Figure 19a).
- Regression analysis showed that binding of insulin glargine to the IGF-1R had only

slightly higher affinity than that of human insulin (half-inhibitory concentrations of 70 and 101 nM, respectively).

- The growth-promoting activity of insulin and insulin glargine, as measured by

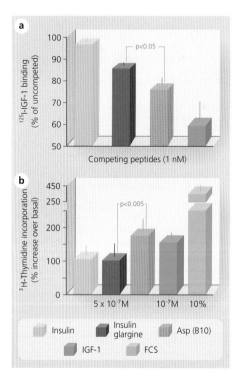

thymidine uptake, were essentially identical with approximately a 2 fold increase in DNA synthesis. In comparison, Asp (B10) caused a greater increase in thymidine uptake (~4 fold) (Figure 19b).

- At lower concentrations, closer to physiologic levels, there was no significant difference in the growth-promoting activities of the three insulins (19-41% over basal).

EDITORS COMMENTARY

The growth-promoting activity and maximal metabolic activity of human insulin and insulin glargine, mediated by IGF-1R in rat muscle cells, are essentially identical. No increased mitogenic effect was evident with insulin glargine in relation to the interaction with the IGF-1R. Other studies examining the interaction of insulin glargine with the insulin receptor have shown normal association and even enhanced disassociation kinetics and unaltered patterns of insulin receptor signaling. Taken together, these findings indicate that the mitogenic potential of insulin glargine is essentially similar to that of human insulin at physiologic concentrations.

Figure 19. (a) Competition of insulin and insulin analogs for [^{125}I]-labeled IGF-1 binding in comparison to unlabeled IGF-1. (b) Effects of insulin, insulin analogs and IGF-1 on [^{3}H]-thymidine incorporation in H9c2 myoblasts. Data are mean values ± S.E.M. (Reprinted from *European Journal of Pharmacology* 1997; 320: 259–265. Reprinted by permission of Elsevier Science B.V..

Additional references

1. Eckel J, Kolter M, Bähr H, Lammerbirt M, Speileken M, Seipke G. Growth promoting and metabolic activity of the insulin analogue HOE 901 in muscle cells. *Diabetologia* 1995; 38(Suppl 1): Abstract 6.

The long acting human insulin analog HOE 901: characteristics of insulin signalling in comparison to Asp (B10) and regular insulin.

Berti L, Kellerer M, Bossenmaier B, Seffer E, Seipke G, Häring HU. *Hormone and Metabolic Research*, 1998; 30:123–129.

In an animal cell line model, insulin glargine behaved like regular human insulin with respect to insulin receptor binding, receptor auto-phosphorylation, phosphorylation of signaling elements and the promotion of mitogenesis in a rat fibroblast cell line over-expressing human insulin receptor A or B isoforms.

STUDY RATIONALE

Insulin analogs, with amino acid substitutions, may alter the normal molecular interaction with the insulin receptor and alter the patterns of intracellular signaling through second messenger pathways. The mode of action of insulin glargine at the molecular level must be characterized and understood. The analog Asp (B10) has a known high mitogenic activity and therefore offers a useful comparator.

OBJECTIVES

To use a cell culture model to study insulin receptor binding and the early intracellular signaling patterns induced by insulin glargine compared to regular human insulin and the rapid-acting insulin analog, Asp (B10).

STUDY DESIGN

An *in vitro* insulin receptor binding and intracellular signaling study undertaken in rat-1 fibroblast cell lines that over-express surface human insulin receptor isoforms A (HIR A) or B (HIR B).

Binding and dissociation

Cells were incubated with [^{125}I]-labeled insulin glargine, human insulin and Asp (B10) at 21°C and the fraction of radioactivity bound by the cells in the presence of the individual ligands was determined by gamma counter at time intervals over a 120 minute period.

Intracellular signaling

Western blotting of whole cell lysates using antibodies to phosphotyrosine and immuno-precipitation with antibodies specific for each of the substrates was used to determine the patterns of phosphorylation and dephosphorylation on the insulin receptor and on intracellular proteins involved in insulin signaling (insulin receptor substrate 1 [IRS-1], insulin receptor substrate 2 [IRS-2] and focal adhesion kinase [p^{125}FAK])

Mitogenic effects were assessed by [^{3}H]-thymidine incorporation into the rat 1 fibroblast cells over-expressing HIR B.

KEY FINDINGS

- Insulin glargine and human insulin showed similar association and dissociation rates with both HIR A and HIR B. Asp (B10) showed a similar association rate as human insulin with both HIR A (Figure 20a) and HIR B (not shown), but a delayed and only partial dissociation from HIR A (Figure 20b) over a period of 120 minutes.

- The three insulins stimulated autophosphorylation of the insulin receptor, but unlike insulin glargine and human insulin, Asp (B10) caused sustained phosphorylation after 60 minutes, with no obvious difference between HIR A (findings shown in Figure 21a) or HIR B.

- In cells stimulated with either insulin glargine or human insulin, similar kinetics of dephosphorylation of the insulin receptor was observed. However, dephosphorylation was delayed in cells stimulated with Asp (B10).

- Similar dephosphorylation kinetics to those observed for the insulin receptor were found for IRS-1 (Figure 21b).

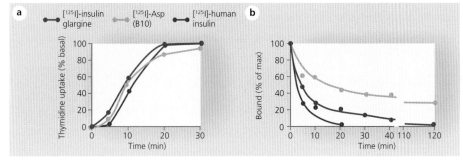

Figure 20. (a) Representative association and (b) dissociation kinetics in rat 1 cells over-expressing HIR A. (Reprinted from *Hormone and Metabolic Research* 1998; 30:123–129. Reprinted with permission from the Thieme Publishing Group).

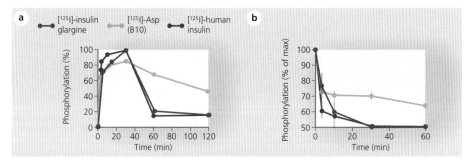

Figure 21. (a) Autophosphorylation kinetics: representative data obtained from laser scanning densitometry in a series of four experiments in rat 1 cells over-expressing HIR A. (b) Dephosphorylation kinetics: representative data obtained from laser scanning densitometry in a series of four experiments ±SE in rat 1 cells over-expressing HIR B. (Reprinted from *Hormone and Metabolic Research* 1998; 30:123–129. Reprinted with permission from the Thieme Publishing Group).

- All three insulins induced dephosphorylation of focal adhesion kinase (p^{125}FAK) with the same efficiency.

- Whereas insulin glargine and human insulin induced [^{3}H]-thymidine incorporation to a similar extent, increased levels of incorporation occurred following stimulation with Asp (B10).

EDITORS COMMENTARY

Insulin glargine behaved in a similar manner to regular human insulin with respect to insulin receptor binding and dissociation kinetics as well as phosphorylation and dephosphorylation of insulin receptor and substrates in the intracellular signaling cascade. Insulin glargine had similar activity to regular human insulin with respect to thymidine uptake, indicating that insulin glargine promotes mitogenesis in a similar way to regular human insulin in contrast to Asp (B10).

Additional references

1. Berti L, Bossenmaier B, Kellerer M, Seffer E, Seipke G, Häring H. Comparison of the human insulin analogs HOE 901 and ASP (B10): characteristics of receptor binding, activation and tyrosine phosphorylation of different substrate proteins. *Diabetologia* 1995; 38(Suppl 1):A191 Abstract 739.

2. Berti L, Seffer E, Seipke G, Kroder G, Häring HU. Human insulin analog HOE901; characteristics of receptor binding and tyrosine kinase activation. *Diabetes* 1995; 44(Suppl 1):243A Abstract 895.

In vitro pharmacology studies with insulin glargine and human insulin: IGF-1 receptor binding and thymidine incorporation.

Sandow J, Seipke G. *Diabetes* **2001; 50(Suppl 1):A429 Abstract 1787–PO.**

Insulin glargine shows low affinity for the IGF-1 receptor and similar levels of mitogenic activity compared to human insulin in the majority of cell lines studied.

STUDY RATIONALE

Alterations in insulin molecular structure can change its interaction not only with the insulin receptor, but also with the structurally homologous insulin-like growth factor-1 (IGF-1R) receptor.

OBJECTIVES

To compare the IGF-1R binding affinity and mitogenic potential of insulin glargine and human insulin with endogenous IGF-1.

STUDY DESIGN

Human hepatoma (HepG2), human osteosarcoma and rat cardiomyoblast cell lines were exposed to [^{125}I]-labeled human insulin, insulin glargine and in some experiments, the analog Asp (B10). A competitive binding assay measured [^{3}H]-thymidine uptake as a surrogate measure of mitogenicity.

KEY FINDINGS

- In human hepatoma HepG2 cells, the affinity for the IGF-1R affinity was 5-7 fold higher for insulin glargine than human insulin, but 300-500 fold lower than that of endogenous IGF-1.
- In human osteosarcoma cells, the IGF-1R affinity of insulin glargine was 3.5-7.6 fold higher than human insulin but 200 fold lower than IGF-1.

- In a second study involving osteosarcoma cells, the affinity of insulin glargine for the IGF-1 receptor was 14 fold higher than human insulin but approximately 2000 fold lower than IGF-1.
- In rat cardiomyoblasts, the IGF-1 receptor affinity was only slightly higher for insulin glargine than human insulin.
- Insulin glargine and human insulin stimulated thymidine uptake in rat cardiomyoblasts to a similar extent. In contrast, the mitogenic activity of the insulin analog, Asp (B10) was significantly higher (p<0.005) and comparable to IGF-1.
- In human osteosarcoma cells, thymidine uptake in response to insulin glargine was 6.1 fold higher than human insulin. Compared to insulin glargine, IGF-1 caused a higher level of thymidine incorporation.

EDITORS COMMENTARY

This series of experiments indicates that *in vitro*, insulin glargine and human insulin have low affinities for the IGF-1R compared to endogenous IGF-1 and that insulin glargine and human insulin stimulate thymidine uptake to a similar extent in the majority of cell lines examined. Although differences between insulin glargine and human insulin-stimulated thymidine uptake were apparent in the osteosarcoma cell line investigated, the increase was only detected at high concentrations that are not expected in the clinical environment.

Effects of the long-acting insulin analog insulin glargine on cultured human skeletal muscle cells: comparisons to insulin and IGF-1.

Ciaraldi TP, Carter L, Seipke G, Mudaliar S, Henry RR. *The Journal of Endocrinology and Metabolism* 2001; 86:5838–5847.

Using a culture system of human skeletal muscle cells derived from healthy subjects and persons with T2DM, insulin glargine behaved with similar activity to human insulin with regard to insulin and IGF-1 receptor binding, and both metabolic and mitogenic responses, including signaling events downstream from the response.

STUDY RATIONALE

The C-terminus of the insulin β chain, which is modified in insulin glargine, is known to significantly influence the interaction with the IGF-1 receptor (IGF-1R). Given that the IGF-1R can mediate growth-promoting effects of ligands other than its cognate hormone, the potentially altered receptor binding characteristics and metabolic and mitogenic responses, including signaling events proximal to these responses, of insulin glargine required detailed investigation.

OBJECTIVES

To compare the metabolic and mitogenic responses to insulin glargine, human insulin and IGF-1 in cultures of differentiated human skeletal muscle cells (HSMC) isolated from both healthy subjects and persons with T2DM.

STUDY DESIGN

A series of *in vitro* insulin and IGF-1R binding, metabolic and mitogenic potency and intracellular signaling studies, comparing human insulin with insulin glargine conducted in HSMC.

Patient cells and culture

HSMC were obtained via muscle biopsies from healthy subjects (n=17) and persons with T2DM (n=16) and were grown in culture and differentiation was induced. Cells were incubated for 4 hours at 12°C with [125I]-labeled insulin (final concentration of 67 pM) or IGF-1 (final concentration of 39 pM) in the absence or presence of varying concentrations of unlabeled regular human insulin, insulin glargine or IGF-1.

Assays

Displacement of labeled insulin or IGF-1 was used to represent binding affinities to HSMC.

Metabolic and mitogenic effects were assessed by measuring glucose uptake (0-methyl glucose) and [3H]-thymidine incorporation respectively.

Intracellular signal transduction was determined by examining the level of intracellular phosphorylation of key proteins in signaling pathways (the serine/threonine kinase, Akt, and MAPK) following stimulation of cells for 15 minutes at 37°C with each of the ligands by Western blotting of cell lysates with antibodies to phosphotyrosine.

KEY FINDINGS

Receptor binding
- Human insulin and insulin glargine were equally potent in their ability to displace bound [125I]-labeled insulin from the insulin receptor, in cells from both healthy persons and those with T2DM.
- Human insulin and insulin glargine had similar affinities for the IGF-1 receptor, except at supra-physiological concentrations. At concentrations of >100 nM, insulin glargine minimally displaced bound [125I]-labeled IGF-1 from its receptor (≈0.5% of the potency of unlabeled IGF-1 (Figure 22).

Metabolic activity – glucose uptake
- All three ligands stimulated glucose uptake similarly in a dose dependent manner in

healthy HSMC. The sensitivity of glucose uptake was greatest in response to IGF-1 and lower but similar for human insulin and insulin glargine.

- Maximum human insulin and insulin glargine stimulated rates of glucose uptake were similar in T2DM cells, but both rates were significantly lower than those in healthy subjects. The maximal response to IGF-1 was greater than that of either human insulin or insulin glargine (Figure 23a and 23b).

Mitogenic activity – thymidine uptake

- Thymidine incorporation into DNA was dose dependent for all three insulin molecules, but the dose-response curves were shifted far to the right for human insulin and insulin glargine, with no significant difference between human insulin and insulin glargine (Figure 24).
- Human insulin and insulin glargine showed equivalent but greatly reduced sensitivities (<1%) compared to IGF-1. Insulin glargine had a lesser effect on thymidine incorporation than human insulin.

Intracellular signaling

- Phosphorylation of Akt was slightly greater in response to IGF-1 compared to human insulin and insulin glargine.
- In cells from healthy subjects, the greatest MAPK phosphorylation was attained after IGF-1 stimulation ($p < 0.05$ vs. insulin glargine and human insulin). Insulin glargine and human insulin were equipotent (Figure 25a and 25b).

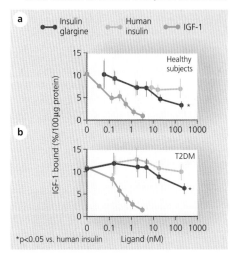

Figure 22. Comparison of affinities for IGF-1 receptor presented as displacement of specific IGF-1 binding, normalized to cell protein in (**a**) cells from normal subjects; (**b**) cells from subjects with T2DM. (Reprinted from *Journal of Clinical Endocrinology & Metabolism* 2001; 86:5838–5847. Reprinted with permission from The Endocrine Society).

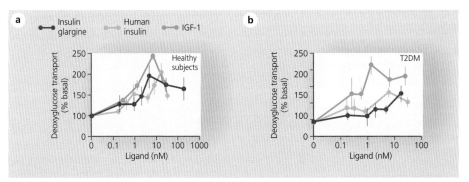

Figure 23. Dose response curves of deoxyglucose uptake calculated as a function of the basal (no added insulin) activity in (**a**) cells from healthy subjects; (**b**) cells from subjects with T2DM. Results are the average ± S.E.M. (Reprinted from *Journal of Clinical Endocrinology & Metabolism* 2001; 86: 5838–5847. Reprinted with permission from The Endocrine Society).

EDITORS COMMENTARY

Overall, these findings indicate that human insulin and insulin glargine are comparable with respect to insulin receptor binding, IGF-1 receptor binding, stimulation of glucose uptake and mitogenic potential.

Insulin glargine displaced human insulin from the insulin receptor with an almost identical efficacy to the native hormone. Although differences between insulin glargine and human insulin were seen with respect to IGF-1 receptor binding, the increase was small and only detected at high concentrations that are not expected in the clinical environment.

In HSMC employed in this study, the mitogenic potential of insulin glargine was not different from human insulin, with both showing elevated mitogenic potential at very high non-physiologic concentration levels.

The use of HSMC has advantages over the system of Saos/B10 human osteosarcoma cells previously described (Kurtzhals et al., 2000; page 39). The relative expression levels of insulin and IGF-1 receptors are similar to skeletal muscle cells *in vivo*, which is the major target for insulin and therefore suggests that this represents a valid physiological model to assess the actions of insulin glargine.

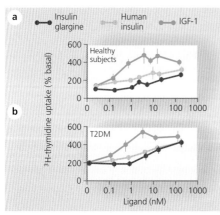

Figure 24. Dose response curves of thymidine uptake into DNA calculated as a function of the basal (no added insulin) activity in (**a**) cells from healthy subjects; (**b**) cells from subjects with T2DM). Results are the average ± S.E.M. (Reprinted from *Journal of Clinical Endocrinology & Metabolism* 2001; 86:5838–5847. Reprinted with permission from The Endocrine Society).

Additional references

1. Ciaraldi TP, Carter L, Mudaliar S, Kim D, Henry RR. Effects of the long acting human analog insulin glargine on cultured human skeletal muscle cells; comparisons with insulin and IGF-1. *Diabetes* 2001; 50(Suppl 2):A417 Abstract 1736–PO.

2. Ciaraldi TP, Carter L, Mudaliar S, Henry RR. Effects of insulin glargine on cultured human skeletal muscle cells: comparisons with insulin and IGF-1. *Diabetologia* 2001; 44(Suppl 1):A160 Abstract 612.

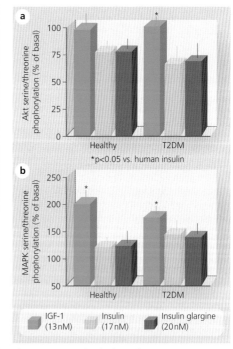

Figure 25. Maximal Akt and MAPK phosphorylation in muscle cells from healthy subjects and subjects with T2DM (n=3-5); results are normalized against the maximal response attained for each individual subject. Results are the average ± S.E.M. (Reprinted from *Journal of Clinical Endocrinology & Metabolism* 2001; 86:5838–5847. Reprinted with permission from The Endocrine Society).

Correlations of receptor binding and metabolic and mitogenic potencies of insulin analogs designed for clinical use.

Kurtzhals P, Chaffer L, Sorensen A, Kristensen C, Jonassen I, Schmid C, Trub T. *Diabetes* 2000; 49:999–1005.

Insulin analogs (including insulin lispro, aspart, glargine and detemir) differ with respect to insulin and IGF-1 receptor binding characteristics and metabolic and mitogenic capacity in *in vitro* cell line models.

STUDY RATIONALE

Previously, an experimental rapid-acting insulin analog, Asp (B10), was shown to cause mammary tumors in female Sprague-Dawley rats. Therefore, as new insulin analogs are introduced into patient care, it is important to define their insulin receptor binding, metabolic and mitogenic characteristics.

OBJECTIVES

To investigate the relationships between insulin structure, insulin receptor and IGF-1 receptor binding characteristics, and the metabolic and mitogenic potency of various insulin analogs (insulin aspart, insulin lispro, insulin glargine and insulin detemir) and other reference insulin analogs.

STUDY DESIGN

A series of *in vitro* insulin receptor binding, metabolic and mitogenic potency studies using hamster, mouse and human cell lines.

Insulin analogs

Insulin aspart, insulin lispro, insulin glargine, insulin detemir, and two analogs containing the component amino acid substitutions present in insulin glargine (A21Gly and B31ArgB32Arg) were studied.

Insulin and IGF-1 receptor binding
- Human insulin receptor (HIR) was isolated from transfected baby hamster kidney (BHK) cells and incubated with [125I]-labeled human insulin (tracer) and various

concentrations of unlabeled human insulin or insulin analogs.
- Bound tracer was estimated and the concentration required for half-maximal effect calculated (EC_{50}). The relative affinity of each analog for the insulin receptor compared to human insulin was calculated from the ratio of EC_{50} values for insulin and individual analogs. IGF-1 receptor affinities were calculated in an analogous manner using purified IGF-1 receptors and [125I]-labeled IGF-1.

Insulin receptor dissociation studies
- Chinese hamster ovary (CHO) cells over expressing HIR were incubated with [125I]-labeled insulins.
- The dissociation of radioactivity was measured following the addition of unlabeled human insulin.
- Cell associated radioactivity was measured as a function of time and dissociation rate constants (K_d) calculated.

Metabolic potency
- Uptake of [3H]-labeled glucose by mouse adipocytes was measured in a dose-response study and EC_{50} determined.
- Relative metabolic potencies were calculated as the ratio of EC_{50} values for human insulin and individual insulin analogs.

Mitogenic potency
- Uptake of [3H]-thymidine in a human osteosarcoma cell line Saos/B10 predominantly expressing IGF-1 receptors was measured.
- Relative mitogenic potency was calculated as the ratio of EC_{50} values for human insulin and individual insulin analogs.

KEY FINDINGS

The insulin and IGF-1 receptor binding properties and metabolic and mitogenic potencies of the series of insulin analogs investigated are detailed below.

Analog	Insulin receptor affinity (%)	Insulin receptor off-rate (%)	Metabolic potency (lipogenesis) (%)	IGF-1 receptor affinity (%)	Mitogenic potency (%)
Human insulin	100	100	100	100	100
Asp (B10)	205 ± 20	14 ± 1	207 ± 14	587 ± 50	975 ± 173
Aspart	92 ± 6	81 ± 8	101 ± 2	81 ± 9	58 ± 22
Lispro	84 ± 6	100 ± 11	82 ± 3	156 ± 16	66 ± 10
Glargine	86 ± 3	152 ± 13	60 ± 3	641 ± 51	783 ± 132
A21Gly	78 ± 10	162 ± 11	88 ± 3	42 ± 11	34 ± 12
B31B32diArg	120 ± 4	75 ± 8	75 ± 5	2,049 ± 202	2,180 ± 390
Detemir	46 ± 5 and 18 ± 2	204 ± 9	ca 27	16 ± 1	ca 11

EDITORS COMMENTARY

This study was conducted using a range of *in vitro* cell line models measuring parameters potentially related to efficacy and safety. In the cell lines studied, the amino acid modifications in the rapid-acting insulin analogs, insulin aspart and insulin lispro, had no significant influence on metabolic and mitogenic potency of human insulin.

Insulin glargine, in these *in vitro* models, exhibited differences compared to human insulin. Relative to human insulin, the affinity of insulin glargine for solubilized insulin receptor was 80-90%, with an off-rate of about 150%. Insulin glargine had a six-fold greater affinity for IGF-1 receptors and an eight-fold greater ability to promote DNA synthesis compared with human insulin in the Saos/B10 osteosarcoma cell line.

This is the only study to demonstrate an increased mitogenic potency of insulin glargine in comparison to human insulin. These results have been assessed and reviewed at length (Kellerer and Häring, 2001). The authors emphasized the very high expression levels (>30,000 per cell) of IGF-1 receptors and the low expression of insulin receptors shift the dose response curves of the Saos/B10 osteosarcoma cell line. With respect to clinical safety implications for insulin glargine, these *in vitro* findings are useful to discriminate which analogs should be investigated further in *in vivo* models, but cannot be necessarily extrapolated to the clinical setting.

Insulin analogues: impact of cell model characteristics on results and conclusions regarding mitogenic properties.

Kellerer M and Häring HU. *Experimental and Clinical Endocrinology and Diabetes* 2001: 109; 63–64.

Two experts reviewed the cell models employed in studies of mitogenic potential of insulin glargine. Certain characteristics of the *in vitro* models employed make it difficult to extrapolate *in vitro* findings to the *in vivo* situation.

STUDY RATIONALE

Numerous studies had analyzed the mitogenic potential of insulin glargine. Two experts reviewed the *in vitro* models that had been employed, in the light of the findings reported by Kurtzhals et al. who had suggested that mitogenic responses to insulin glargine may be a cause for concern.

OBJECTIVES

To compare the features and characteristics of the *in vitro* models used previously to assess mitogenic potential in studies of insulin glargine.

STUDIES AND CELL LINES REVIEWED

The studies by Bähr et al. (1997) of rat cardiac myoblasts and ventricular cardiomyocytes (page 31), Berti et al. (1998) of transfected rat-1 fibroblasts (page 33) and Kurtzhals et al. (2000) of human osteosarcoma cell lines (page 39).

KEY FINDINGS

- Bahr et al. had found no increased mitogenic potential in rat cardiac myoblasts and ventricular cardiomyocytes expressing low levels of insulin and IGF-1R.

- Berti et al. found in rat-1 HIR fibroblasts, a cell line model thought optimal to assess mitogenic potential of insulin analogs and which expresses high levels of insulin receptor and low levels of IGF-1R, no increased mitogenic potential.

- Features of the human osteosarcoma cell line Saos-B10 impact on the cell lines behavior and on how mitogenic results should be interpreted.

- The high levels of IGF-1R (>30000 per cell) and low levels of insulin receptor (<1000) make it likely that all insulin receptors exist as insulin/IGF-1R hybrid proteins, thus excluding the effect of any binding to endogenous insulin receptors in experiments with Saos-B10 cells.

- Regular insulin binds to IGF-1R with a 1000 fold lower affinity, but the ED_{50} for mitogenic stimulation differs only 80-fold in Saos-B10 cells, suggesting differences in IGF-1R make-up compared with the normal human IGF-1R.

- Overall, the ED_{50} for mitogenic stimulation in Saos-B10 cells for IGF-1 is much lower than in other cell models, confirming that dose response curves for mitogenic potential are altered by each particular cell line's characteristics.

EDITORS COMMENTARY

This review indicates that the cell lines used to assess the mitogenic potential of insulin glargine have different features which impact significantly on how the *in vitro* findings can be interpreted and potentially translated to assessments of the *in vivo* situation. The expert commentary concludes that it would be inappropriate to assign any message regarding mitogenic potential to insulin glargine therapy from the published findings.

Insulin-like growth factor 1 receptors are more abundant than insulin receptors in human micro- and macrovascular endothelial cells

Chisalita SI, Arnqvist HJ. American Journal of Physiology Endocrinology and Metabolism. 2004; 286:E896–901.

Human endothelial cells express insulin receptor and functioning IGF-I receptors; insulin glargine had a higher affinity for the IGF-I receptor in human coronary artery endothelial cells than human insulin, but this had no effect on DNA synthesis, even at high concentrations.

STUDY RATIONALE

Endothelial cell dysfunction is thought to play an important role in the process of diabetes-related micro- and macroangiopathy. There is, however, little information on insulin receptor (IR) and insulin-like growth factor 1 receptor (IGF-1R) expression in human endothelial cells or on the biological effect of human insulin and insulin analogs binding at these receptors.

OBJECTIVES

To characterize IR and IGF-1R receptor gene expression, ligand binding and receptor activation characteristics, and to examine the biological effect of IGF-1, human insulin and insulin glargine *in vitro* on human dermal microvascular endothelial cells (HMVEC) and human aortic (macrovascular) endothelial cells (HAEC).

STUDY DESIGN

IR and IGF-1R gene expression, receptor binding and phosphorylation, metabolic and mitogenic potency studies were conducted, comparing the effects of IGF-1, human insulin and insulin glargine in human endothelial cells *in vitro*.

Commercial cultures of HMVEC and HAEC were grown under standard conditions. The mRNA expression of the IR and IGF-1R genes was determined by quantitative real-time RT-PCR. Ligand binding by receptors was determined using [125 I]-labelled insulin and [125 I]-IGF-1. Receptor phosphorylation was determined by immunoprecipitation and

Western blotting. DNA synthesis and glucose incorporation was quantified by measuring [3 H]-thymidine and [3 H]-glucose incorporation, respectively, into HMVEC cells only. Findings are presented as means ± SE.

KEY FINDINGS

- Gene expression of IR and IGF-1R was demonstrated in HMVEC and HAEC. IGF-1R was expressed at significantly higher levels (5-8 fold) compared to IR (p<0.001).
- Specific binding of [125I]-IGF-1 to HMVEC was 1.6 ± 0.2% of the total [125I]-IGF-1 added, which fits a one-site binding model. The concentration of unlabeled ligand required for half-maximal displacement (EC_{50}) was 5.7×10^{-10} M for IGF-1, 2.2×10^{-7} M for insulin and 2.5×10^{-8} M for insulin glargine.
- The specific binding of [125I]-IGF-1 in HAEC was 1.9 ± 0.1% of the total [125I]-IGF-1 added. EC_{50} was 4.3×10^{-10} M for unlabeled IGF-1, 5.8×10^{-6} M for insulin and for insulin glargine, 9.9×10^{-8} M.
- The specific binding of [125 I]-insulin was lower than [125 I]-IGF-1 in both cell types (0.5 ± 0.2% in HMVEC and 0.2 ± 0.04% in HAEC).
- The β subunit of the IGF-IR was phosphorylated by IGF-1 at a concentration of 10^{-8} M in HMVEC and HAEC. A much higher insulin concentration (10^{-6} M) was required for phosphorylation in HAEC. In HMVEC, IGF-1R was phosphorylated by insulin glargine at concentrations of 10^{-6} M and weakly at 10^{-8} M.
- The incorporation of [3 H]-thymidine into DNA of HMVEC was highly significant at 10^{-7} M concentration of IGF-1 (P < 0.002),

with no effect with either insulin or insulin glargine.

- IGF-1 significantly stimulated glucose incorporation at 10^{-7} M ($P = 0.008$), 10^{-8} M ($P = 0.02$), and 10^{-9} M ($P = 0.009$); there was no effect evident with either insulin or insulin glargine.

Additional references

1. Chisalita SI, Arnqvist HJ. IGF-1 receptors are more expressed than insulin receptors in human coronary artery endothelial cells. *Diabetes Metabolism* 2003; 29(Spec No 2):Abstract 1191.

EDITORS COMMENTARY

These *in vitro* studies show that micro- and macrovascular cell lines express IGF-1R and IR that bind ligand, with a higher population of IGF-1R present. The binding studies showed that insulin was approximately a thousand-fold less potent, and with insulin glargine a hundred-fold less potent, than IGF-1 at displacing [^{125}I]-IGF-1 from its receptor. This represents a 10-fold difference between human insulin and insulin glargine with regard to affinity for the IGF-1 receptor in HMVEC. Phosphorylation of the IGF-1 receptor was achieved at a higher concentration (10^{-6} M) of both insulin and insulin glargine compared to IGF-1 (10^{-8} M) in HMVEC and HAEC. There was no mitogenic or metabolic effect of both insulin and insulin glargine, whereas IGF-1 increased both significantly at higher concentrations of 10^{-7} M.

Toxicology

Evaluation of the reproductive toxicity and embryotoxicity of insulin glargine (LANTUS) in rats and rabbits.

Hofmann T, Horstmann G, Stammberger I. *International Journal of Toxicology* 2002; 21:181–189.

In rats, insulin glargine has no adverse effects on reproduction, embryofetal and post-natal development. In rabbits, maternal and embryofetal toxicity was related to the hypoglycemic effect of the insulin.

STUDY RATIONALE

Before treating women with DM who are, or are planning to become pregnant, with novel insulin analogs, such as insulin glargine, careful safety evaluation is required. Animal studies were therefore undertaken to explore the effect of insulin glargine on reproduction, the embryo and the fetus.

OBJECTIVES

To determine the effect of daily subcutaneous administration of insulin glargine and NPH insulin on reproduction and/or embryofetal development in rats and rabbits.

STUDY DESIGN

The impact of varying doses of insulin glargine on reproduction in rats and on embryo development in rats and rabbits was compared to findings with both NPH insulin and a control solution.

The study was conducted in compliance with the European Community guideline III/3387/93 'Detection of toxicity to reproduction for medicinal products.' Insulin glargine was diluted in a control aqueous solution containing zinc at pH 4.0. NPH insulin was diluted in an aqueous solution at pH 7.3. The vehicle control solution was an aqueous solution at pH 4.0. Reproductive toxicity and embryotoxicity were assessed in Wistar rats and additionally, embryotoxicity was assessed in previously virginal Himalayan rabbits.

Reproductive toxicity

Rats (25 male, 25 female) received daily subcutaneous injections of insulin glargine (1, 3 or 10 U/kg), NPH insulin (3 U/kg) or a control solution during the pre-mating and mating periods (males and females), throughout pregnancy (females) and 21-day lactation period (females). The lowest dose of insulin glargine was approximately twice the maximal therapeutic dose used in humans (0.5-1.0 U/kg). Effects on reproduction were assessed by measuring sperm motility in male rats and by monitoring the normal development of pups grown to maturity.

Embryotoxicity

Female rats (20 per group) were given daily subcutaneous injections of insulin glargine (2, 6.3 or 20 U/kg), NPH insulin (6.3 U/kg) or a control solution between days 7-18 of pregnancy. The lowest dose of insulin glargine was approximately twice the anticipated maximal therapeutic dose used in humans (0.5-1.0 U/kg).

Female rabbits (n=20) were treated with insulin glargine (0.5, 1.0 or 2.0 U/kg) or NPH insulin (1 U/kg) between days 6-18 of pregnancy. The range of insulin glargine doses used was based on the range at which no signs of maternal or embryofetal toxicity were expected and where signs of intolerance in the parental animals and conceptuses were expected. Embryotoxicity was assessed by sacrificing pregnant females on the 21st and 29th day after mating and examining fetuses for abnormalities.

KEY FINDINGS

Reproductive toxicity

- Treatment with insulin glargine or NPH insulin led to a dose-dependent hypoglycemic response with respect to degree and duration.
- Hypoglycemia in the groups of rats receiving 1 or 3 U/kg insulin glargine did not result in clinical signs and no impairment in behavior or general condition was observed.
- In the group receiving 10 U/kg insulin glargine, 5 female rats died or were killed. These events were though to be caused by hypoglycemic shock. In the remaining rats, no adverse effects on physical condition, fertility, course of pregnancy, parturition, or the post-natal development of off-spring were observed.
- The physical development, sensory functions, sexual maturation, behavior and fertility of off-spring were unaffected by insulin administration.
- Sperm motility was unaffected by administration of insulin glargine or NPH insulin.
- Autopsy of parent animals and their offspring showed no detrimental effects of insulin glargine or NPH insulin on internal organs.

Embryotoxicity

- In rats, insulin glargine and NPH insulin had no effect on pregnancy, intrauterine death rate or intrauterine development.
- Morphological, cross-section and skeletal examinations of rat fetuses revealed no malformations, abnormalities or developmental retardation that was considered to be compound-induced.
- In rabbits, administration of insulin glargine or NPH insulin resulted in dose-dependent hypoglycemia with respect to severity and duration.

- No impairment of behavior or general condition was observed in the groups of rabbits receiving 0.5 or 1.0 U/kg insulin glargine. However, two animals in the 2.0 U/kg group and one in the NPH insulin group developed hypoglycemic shock and died or were killed.
- In the group of rabbits receiving 0.5 U/kg insulin glargine, pregnancy and intrauterine development were unaffected by treatment.
- In the groups of rabbits receiving 1.0 or 2.0 U/kg insulin glargine there was a dose-dependent increase in abortion, or dead fetuses with an increase in early intrauterine death in the 2.0 U/kg group. In the NPH insulin group, there was an increase in the rates of abortion and early intrauterine death.
- At the highest insulin glargine dose, compound-dependent changes in the fetuses included a slight increase in ventricular dilation of the brain and of blood in the thoracic cavity.

EDITORS COMMENTARY

Apart from toxicologic effects induced by hypoglycemia, insulin glargine had no independent effect on the reproduction, embryonic development and post-natal development in rats. Rabbits, however, proved to be more sensitive to hypoglycemia with increased rates of abortion, dead fetuses and early intrauterine death related to the insulin dose. The results from this study show that any apparent effect of insulin glargine on reproduction and embryology in rats and rabbits is due to hypoglycemia and not any toxic effects of insulin glargine itself. Of note, insulin glargine is not approved for use in human pregnancy.

Evaluation of the carcinogenic potential of insulin glargine (LANTUS) in rats and mice.

Stammberger I, Bube A, Durchfeld-Meyer B, Donaubauer H, Troschau G. *International Journal of Toxicology* 2002; 21:171–179.

> Insulin glargine did not exhibit a systemic carcinogenic effect in mice or rats after exposure over a two year period.

STUDY RATIONALE

Careful assessments are needed of the mitogenic and carcinogenic potential of modified insulins before clinical administration. Several cell lines have been used to assess the mitogenicity of insulin glargine, but there was a need to assess the carcinogenic potential of insulin glargine using *in vivo* models.

OBJECTIVES

To determine if insulin glargine has any carcinogenic potential by conducting studies in rodents (NMRI mice and Sprague - Dowley rats) over a two year duration.

STUDY DESIGN

> General toxicity studies, followed by carcinogenic studies in mice and rats using a range of doses of insulin glargine including NPH insulin for comparison with saline and vehicle as control.

Mice (10 male and 10 female), (NMRI species) received daily subcutaneous injections of 5, 10 and 20 U/kg of insulin glargine and general toxicity was assessed at 3 and 6 months. Based on these results, 2 year carcinogenicity studies were performed using mice (50 of each sex) and rats (Sprague - Dowley, 50 of each sex).

The animals received over the 2 year period once daily subcutaneous injections of either vehicle solution (control), saline (control), insulin glargine (2.5 or 12.5 U/kg) or

NPH insulin (12.5 U/kg in mice and 5 U/kg in rats) for comparative purposes.

The lowest dose used in the carcinogenicity studies was approximately two-times higher than the maximal therapeutic dose used in humans (0.5 - 1.0 U/kg). Health and survival checks were conducted frequently. Hematology parameters were measured and necropsy examinations conducted.

KEY FINDINGS

• In mice, the mortality rate over the 2 year study was comparable between the treatment groups.

• Mortality rates in male rats showed a significant increase in animals treated with vehicle solution, insulin glargine and NPH insulin, compared to saline treated control animals ($p<0.05$). In female rats a significant increase in mortality was only observed in animals receiving the highest dose of insulin glargine and NPH insulin, compared to control animals.

• There was no increased incidence of mammary tumors in both mice (table 2) and rats (table 3) in the insulin glargine-treated groups compared with saline control and NPH insulin-treated groups.

• Malignant fibrous histiocytoma (MFH) at the injection site were found in significantly greater numbers in the insulin glargine-treated (2 U/kg) male mice and in the vehicle and all insulin glargine-treated male rats. This effect was not dose dependent.

Test	Dose (U/Kg/d)	Duration (months)	Mammary tumors (n) Benign	Malignant
Saline control	0	24	2	0
Vehicle	0	24	0	0
Insulin glargine	2	24	0	0
	5	24	0	0
	12.5	24	2	0
NPH insulin	12.5	24	2	1

Table 2. Incidence of mammary tumors in female mice in a 2-year carcinogenicity study.

Test	Dose (U/Kg/d)	Duration (months)	Adenoma	Adeno-carcinoma	Fibro-adenoma	Carcinoma*	Mixed malignant
Saline control	0	24	0	9	26	3	0
Vehicle	0	24	1	9	21	2	2
Insulin glargine	2	24	3	7	26	1	0
	5	24	0	8	22	1	0
	12.5	24	0	7	15**	2	0
NPH insulin	5	24	1	7	28	2	0

*Adenocarcinoma arising in fibroadenoma   **$p<0.05$ compared with the NaCl control

Table 3. Incidence of mammary tumors in female rats in the 2-year carcinogenicity study.

EDITORS COMMENTARY

Unlike the findings previously with the insulin analog, Asp (B10), no increased systemic carcinogenicity was observed with insulin glargine over a 2-year period of exposure. Although hepatocellular adenomas and carcinomas were found in mice, these are tumors which are commonly found. The MFH described at the injection site are a recognized phenomenon in laboratory rodents, and are considered to be a result of the local inflammatory reaction.

Additional references

1. Stammberger I, Troschau G, Donaubauer H. Insulin glargine is not carcinogenic in rats and mice. *Diabetes* 2001; 50(Suppl 2):A429 Abstract 1788–PO.

Abstract

Mixture of regular human insulin and insulin glargine injected subcutaneously in healthy dogs does not increase risk of hypoglycaemia.

Werner U, Gerlach M, Hofmann M, Seipke G. *Diabetes* 2002; 51(Suppl 2): A269 Abstract 1205-P.

The subcutaneous administration of a mixture of insulin glargine and regular human insulin did not result in any safety hazard in dogs.

STUDY RATIONALE

The modifications introduced to the human insulin amino acid sequence to produce insulin glargine alter the isoelectric point, resulting in insolubility at physiologic pH. Mixing insulin glargine with regular human insulin is not recommended. This study investigated if inadvertent mixing of the two insulins would present a safety hazard.

OBJECTIVES

To compare the glucose-lowering effect of a mixture of insulin glargine and regular insulin after subcutaneous injection in dogs.

STUDY DESIGN

Insulin glargine and regular insulin were administered to healthy dogs as a mixture, as separate injections or individually. Blood glucose levels were monitored over 24 hours.

Healthy, male, fasted, beagle dogs (n=56) were randomized to one of four groups and received subcutaneous injections of insulin or insulin mixtures. The groups were:

1. A mixture of pre-mixed regular insulin (0.1 U/kg) and insulin glargine (0.1 U/kg)
2. Single injections of regular human insulin (0.1 U/kg) and insulin glargine (0.1 U/kg)
3. Regular human insulin (0.2 U/kg)
4. Insulin glargine (0.2 U/kg)

Blood glucose levels were determined before injection and at a series of time points over 24

hours. Hypoglycemia was defined as a blood glucose level of < 40 mg/dL (2.22 mmol/L).

KEY FINDINGS

- No episodes of severe hypoglycemia occurred in any animal in each of the four treatment groups.
- The incidence of hypoglycemia was highest with regular human insulin only (group 3, 9/14 dogs).
- Groups 1, 2, and 3 were each characterized by a rapid onset of insulin action that had similar glucose lowering effects, reflecting the activity of the regular human insulin.
- In contrast, group 4 had a different profile with delayed, but sustained, effectiveness and a significantly lower nadir.

EDITORS COMMENTARY

This study provides useful safety data on the effect of inadvertent mixing and subsequent administration of insulin glargine and regular human insulin. Mixing insulin glargine with other insulins is not recommended due to the sensitivity of insulin glargine to changes in pH. The study, conducted in dogs, suggests that inadvertent mixing would not constitute a safety hazard. In reality, mixing of the two insulins resulted in similar glucose-lowering effects, but the formation of a milky precipitate should alert users to realize that mixing was inappropriate.

CLINICAL PHARMACOLOGY STUDIES

Pharmacokinetic, pharmacodynamic and metabolic studies

Comparison of the pharmacokinetics/dynamics of GLY(A21)-ARG(B31,B32)- human-insulin (HOE71GT) with NPH-insulin following subcutaneous injection by using euglycaemic clamp technique.

Dreyer M, Pein M, Schmidt Chr, Heidtmann B, Schlunzen M, Rosskamp R. *Diabetologia* 1994; 37(Suppl 1):A87 Abstract 303.

Abstract

Early formulations of insulin glargine (HOE71GT) showed prolonged action and less pronounced peaks of insulin action compared to NPH insulin in healthy subjects.

STUDY RATIONALE

When this study was presented in 1994, research was ongoing to find a new insulin that would satisfy the requirement for a long acting basal insulin. This study set out to investigate the time-action profile of a new, potentially long-acting insulin analog (HOE71GT), later to be developed and known as HOE901 and then insulin glargine.

OBJECTIVES

To compare the time-action characteristics (pharmacodynamics) of a subcutaneous injection of two formulations of HOE71GT differing in their zinc content with NPH insulin in healthy subjects over a 24 hour period, post administration.

STUDY DESIGN

Randomized, double-blind, cross-over trial using the 'euglycemic' clamp technique conducted over a 24 hour period using somatostatin suppression of endogenous insulin secretion comparing NPH insulin and HOE71GT (15 µg/ml zinc or 80 µg/ml zinc).

In a randomized, double-blind, crossover design, HOE901 with either 15 or 80 µg/ml zinc was injected in 12 healthy male subjects. On each study day, subjects received a single subcutaneous injection of either HOE71GT or NPH insulin at a dose of 0.2 U/kg body weight. Somatostatin was given intravenously to suppress exogenous insulin secretion and C-peptide secretion was suppressed during the entire clamp period of 24 hours.

KEY FINDINGS

- The mean time point of the maximum insulin action, as determined by the glucose infusion rate, was significantly delayed with HOE71GT compared to NPH insulin (12.13 ± 3.75 hours [HOE 71GT-15] and 12.98 ± 4.75 hours [HOE 71GT-80] vs. 6.54 ± 2.92 hours, respectively; p<0.01).
- The maximal action of insulin (mg kg. min) was significantly lower for both analogs (2.14 ± 0.75 [HOE 71GT-15] and 1.90 ± 0.62 [HOE71GT-80] vs. 4.02 ± 2.22, respectively; p<0.01).
- The duration of insulin action was longer than 24 hours for both formulations of HOE 71GT compared to NPH insulin (16.22 ± 1.45 hours) (Figure 26).

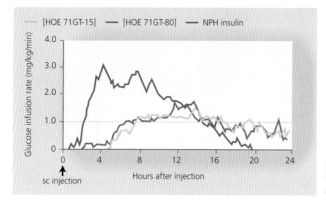

Figure 26. Time action profiles based on glucose infusion rates after subcutaneous injection.

EDITORS COMMENTARY

This "euglycemic" clamp study was one of the earliest research studies published in the development program of insulin glargine (reviewed by Rosskamp and Park, 1999). The study was performed to characterize the action profile over 24 hours after subcutaneous injection at the abdominal site of two early formulations of insulin glargine (HOE71GT), which differed in their zinc content. Previous X-ray crystallography studies had shown that the changes to the amino acid sequence altered the association properties, making the hexamer structure more stable (Hilgenfeld et al., 1992). In animal models, the addition of small amounts of zinc had further prolonged the duration of action and therefore early human studies had used different zinc content. The median glucose infusion rate is shown in Figure 15. NPH insulin showed a characteristic profile, achieving its maximum effect after 5 hours and decreasing in activity from 10 hours. In contrast, HOE71GT was characterized by a longer duration of action over the 24-hour clamp period with a constant peakless profile of insulin action compared to NPH insulin, irrespective of the zinc content of the formulation. These features suggested that insulin glargine may be suitable for providing basal insulin requirements in persons with DM and that further research was warranted.

References

1. Rosskamp R and Park G. Long-Acting Insulin Analogs. *Diabetes Care* 1999; 22(Suppl 2): B109–B113.

2. Hilgenfeld R, Dörschug M, Geisen K, Neubauer H, Obermeier R, Seipke G, Berchtold H: Controlling insulin bioavailability by crystal contact engineering. *Diabetologia* 1992; 35(Suppl 1):A193.

Pharmacokinetics of ^{125}I-labelled insulin glargine (HOE 901) in healthy men.

Owens DR, Coates PA, Luzio SD, Tinbergen JP, Kurzhals R. *Diabetes Care* 2000; 23:813–819.

Insulin glargine exhibits prolonged absorption from the subcutaneous site of injection in healthy subjects, with the same rate of absorption irrespective of injection site.

STUDY RATIONALE

In early studies insulin glargine was formulated with different zinc concentrations. There was a need to assess the subcutaneous absorption of formulations containing 15 or 80 µg/ml of zinc and to examine if site of injection altered the absorption characteristics.

OBJECTIVES

Study one
To compare the absorption rates from subcutaneous tissue and the appearance in plasma of two formulations of insulin glargine (containing 15 or 80 µg/ml zinc) to NPH insulin.

Study two
To examine the influence of the site of subcutaneous injection on the absorption of insulin glargine (containing 30 µg/ml zinc).

STUDY DESIGN

Randomized, single center, crossover studies, single-blinded (study one) or unblinded (study two) in healthy male subjects using [^{125}I]-radio-labeled insulins and external gamma radiation counting to define the rate of absorption from the subcutaneous site of injection.

The rate of absorption from subcutaneous tissue was determined from levels of residual radioactivity following injection of [^{125}I]-labeled insulin (at residue A14). Residual radioactivity was determined over time by placing a gamma counter 50mm from the subcutaneous injection site and the radioactivity counted for periods of 5 minutes, over the 24 hour post-injection period.

The primary pharmacokinetic endpoint was the time in hours for 25% of the administered radioactivity to disappear ($T_{75}\%$). The appearance of (exogenous) insulin in plasma was estimated from measurements of immunoreactive insulin and C-peptide concentrations in plasma.

Study one
Insulins (0.15 U/kg) and placebo were administered by subcutaneous injection into the abdominal wall in 12 healthy male volunteers on four study days, separated by washout periods of >7days.

Study two
Absorption of insulins were determined following subcutaneous injection into the anterior abdominal wall, arm or thigh in 12 healthy male subjects on three study days, separated by washout periods of 7-14 days.

KEY FINDINGS

Study one
- Mean $T_{75}\%$ for NPH insulin was significantly shorter compared to insulin glargine [15] or insulin glargine [80] (3.21 vs. 8.75 vs. 11.01 hours, respectively, p<0.0001).
- Mean residual radioactivity after 24 hours was lower for NPH insulin compared to insulin glargine [15] or insulin glargine [80] (21.90 ± 9.85% vs. 43.84 ± 15.04% vs. 52.17 ±

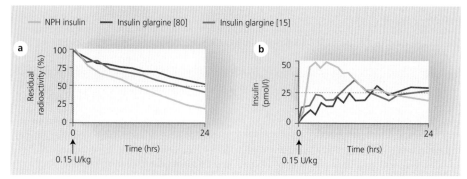

Figure 27. (**a**) Comparison of median percentage residual radioactivity over 24 hours. (**b**) Comparison of plasma exogenous insulin levels. ©2000 American Diabetes Association. *Diabetes Care* 2000; 23:813–819. Reprinted with permission.

15.84%, respectively, p<0.0001) (Figure 27a).
- Plasma exogenous insulin levels between 0-6 hours were significantly higher with NPH insulin compared to insulin glargine [15] and insulin glargine [80] (6.69 ± 4.34 vs. 3.14 ± 1.91 vs. 2.95 ± 2.59 mU/L, respectively, p=0.0017) (Figure 27b).
- The blood glucose levels over 0-6 hours after insulin administration were significantly lower for NPH insulin compared with glargine [15] and [80] (4.84 ± 0.61 vs. 5.17 ± 0.42 vs. 5.28 ± 0.34 respectively; p<0.001.

Study two
- No significant differences in the absorption of insulin glargine [30] at the three injection sites were found, as shown by $T_{75}\%$ (hours): arm (11.9 ± 6.2), thigh (15.3 ± 6.2) and abdomen (13.2 ± 4.6) (Figure 28a) and residual radioactivity (after 24 hours): arm (47.7 ± 17.9 %), thigh (56.3 ± 14.8 %) and abdomen (57.2 ± 16.0 %).
- Comparing the three injection sites, no significant differences in exogenous plasma insulin concentrations (Figure 28b) or plasma glucose levels were found.

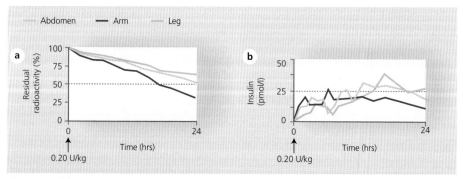

Figure 28. (**a**) Comparison of median percentage residual radioactivity over 24 hours. (**b**) Comparison of plasma exogenous insulin levels. ©2000 American Diabetes Association. *Diabetes Care* 2000; 23:813–819. Reprinted with permission.

EDITORS COMMENTARY

The subcutaneous absorption of insulin glargine was clearly prolonged compared to NPH insulin. The exogenous plasma insulin profiles demonstrated a peak with NPH insulin at 3-5 hours, compared with a slower absorption and relatively peakless plasma insulin profile for both formulations of insulin glargine. The approximate time to disappearance of 50% radioactivity from the abdominal wall injection site (T_{50}%) for insulin glargine from the two studies was around 24 hours compared to 11 hours with NPH insulin.

There was little or no difference in the rate of absorption of insulin glargine between the main subcutaneous injection sites – an important fact to establish before widespread clinical usage. These studies provide clear evidence that insulin glargine is absorbed from the subcutaneous tissue at approximately half the rate of the 'intermediate – acting' NPH insulin suggesting insulin glargine is better suited as a basal insulin.

Additional references

1. Owens D, Luzio S, Tinbergen J, Kurzhals R. The absorption of HOE 901 in healthy subjects. *Diabetologia* 1998; 41(Suppl 1):A245 Abstract 949.

2. Owens D, Luzio S, Beck P, Coates P, Tinbergen J, Kurzhals R. The absorption of insulin analogue HOE 901 from different sites in healthy subjects. *Diabetes* 1997; 46(Suppl 1):329A Abstract 1255.

3. Coates PA, Mukherjee S, Luzio S, Srodzinski KA, Kurzhals KA, Roskamp R, Owens DR. Pharmacokinetics of a 'long-acting' human insulin analogue (HOE901) in healthy subjects. *Diabetes* 1995; 44 (Suppl 1):130A Abstract 478.

Time-action profile of the long-acting insulin analog insulin glargine (HOE901) in comparison with those of NPH insulin and placebo.

Heinemann L, Linkeschova R, Rave K, Hompesch B, Sedlak M, Heise T. *Diabetes Care* 2000; 23:644–649.

Insulin glargine has a peakless time-action profile that lasts 24 hours, whereas NPH insulin has a distinct peak with a shorter duration of action.

STUDY RATIONALE

The time-action profile of insulin glargine (zinc concentration of 30µg/ml) had not been compared to NPH insulin in healthy volunteers using a euglycemic glucose clamp technique. Therefore, a clinical study was conducted to fully characterize the insulin glargine-associated glucose lowering effect.

OBJECTIVES

To compare the time-action pharmacodynamic profile of a subcutaneous injection of insulin glargine and NPH insulin in healthy, subjects over a 30 hour period, post administration.

STUDY DESIGN

Randomized, double-blind, placebo-controlled, 3-way cross-over, 'euglycemic' glucose clamp study.

Subjects, timing and medication

Healthy male volunteers (age 27 ± 4 years with BMI 22.2 ± 1.8 kg/m^2 and insulin antibody negative) received a single subcutaneous injection of insulin glargine, NPH insulin or placebo on one of three study days in random order, with a washout period of 7 days between the study days.

'Euglycemic' glucose clamp

Each study day required the subjects to have fasted overnight. They were connected to a Biostator and a 'euglycemic' glucose clamp was established using a constant intravenous infusion of insulin (0.15 mU/kg/min) and a variable glucose infusion rate. After a baseline period of 2 hours, subjects received a subcutaneous injection of insulin glargine, NPH insulin (0.4 U/kg) or placebo. Glucose infusion rates (GIRs) were established to maintain blood glucose levels at 90 mg/dL (5 mmol/L) over the 30 hour post-administration period. Blood samples were collected every 30 minutes to determine blood glucose levels and every 60 minutes to determine serum insulin and serum C-peptide levels.

KEY FINDINGS

- The hypoglycemic activity (reflected in the GIR) of insulin glargine increased slowly to a plateau level after 4 hours and remained relatively constant for the remainder of the observation period (30 hours) (Figure 29).
- NPH insulin required a pronounced peak in glucose infusion approximately 4-6 hours after injection, followed by a steady decline over the remainder of the study period.
- The maximal hypoglycemic activity (GIR$_{max}$) observed with insulin glargine was lower and occurred later (t$_{max}$) compared to NPH insulin (GIR: 5.3 ± 1.1 vs. 7.7 ± 1.3 mg/kg/min, p<0.05 and (t$_{max}$) 8.6 ± 4.4 vs. 5.4 ± 1.0 hours, p<0.01).
- Similarly, total metabolic activity (AUC 0-30 hours) was lower with insulin glargine compared to NPH insulin (7.92 ± 1.82 vs. 9.24 ± 1.29 g/kg, p<0.05).

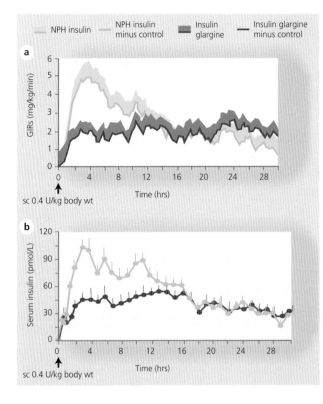

NPH insulin — NPH insulin minus control — Insulin glargine — Insulin glargine minus control

Figure 29. (a) Glucose infusion rates after subcutaneous injection after subtraction of the metabolic effect observed in the control experiments with placebo. (b) Serum insulin concentrations after subcutaneous injection after correction for the serum insulin levels observed in the control experiments with placebo. Data are means ± S.E.M. ©2000 American Diabetes Association. *Diabetes Care* 2000; 23:644–649. Reprinted with permission.

EDITORS COMMENTARY

This well designed study was conducted as a randomized, placebo controlled trial utilizing the euglycemic glucose clamp, to determine the time- action characteristics of insulin glargine and NPH insulin. The placebo arm ensured that the metabolic effect i.e. the glucose requirements elicited by constant basal insulin infusion used, was known under these conditions. It is reasonable to assume that the time action profiles measured are predictive of those in persons with DM.

This study shows that the activities of insulin glargine increased to a plateau within 4 hours. Insulin glargine showed a smooth, peakless time-action profile that lasted more than 24 hours, whereas NPH insulin had a distinct peak 4-7 hours after injection. These characteristics suggest insulin glargine may be suitable for supplying basal insulin as a once daily, subcutaneous injection.

Additional references

1. Rave K, Heise T, Heinemann L. Time-action profile of insulin glargine (HOE901) in Japanese volunteers. *Diabetes* 2000; 49(Suppl 1):A363 Abstract 1524–PO.

2. Rave K, Heinemann L, Rosenkranz B, Heise T. Time-action profile of insulin glargine (HOE901) in Japanese volunteers. *Experimental and Clinical Endocrinology and Diabetes* 2000; 108(Suppl 1): S161 Abstract pFr116.

3. Linkeschova R, Heise T, Rave K, Hompesch B, Heinemann L. Time-action profile of the long-acting insulin analogue HOE901. *Diabetologia* 1999; 42(Suppl 1):A234 Abstract 880.

4. Linkeschova R, Heise T, Rave K, Hompesch B, Sedlack M, Heinemann L. Time-action profile of the long-acting insulin analogue HOE901. *Diabetes* 1999; 48(Suppl 1);A97 Abstract 0417.

5. Linkeschova R, Rave R, Heise T, Hompesch B, Sedlak M, Heinemann L. Wirkprofil des langwirkenden insulin–analogons HOE901. *Diabetes und Stoffwechsel* 1999; 8(Suppl 1):Abstract A55.

Comparison of subcutaneous absorption of insulin glargine (Lantus®) and NPH insulin in patients with type 2 diabetes.

Luzio SD, Beck P, Owens DR. *Hormone and Metabolic Research* 2003; 35:434–438.

> Insulin glargine has a longer presence in subcutaneous tissue with much slower absorption profile compared to NPH insulin, resulting in improved insulin supply.

STUDY RATIONALE

Previous studies in healthy subjects had shown that insulin glargine exhibits delayed absorption characteristics compared to NPH insulin, but there was a need to examine these findings in persons with T2DM.

OBJECTIVES

To compare the subcutaneous absorption characteristics of insulin glargine to NPH insulin in persons with T2DM.

STUDY DESIGN

> An insulin glargine pharmacokinetic study with a randomized two-way cross-over design in insulin-naïve persons with T2DM comparing [^{125}I]-radiolabeled NPH insulin and insulin glargine using external gamma radiation measurement.

Insulin-naïve persons (n=14) with T2DM (age 40-70 years, BMI <30 kg/m^2, HbA$_{1c}$ <10%, and 10 treated with OHA) were administered, by subcutaneous injection into the anterior abdominal wall, NPH insulin glargine or insulin (0.3 U/kg), [^{125}I]-radiolabeled at residue A14, on two study days, separated by washout periods of >7days. After insulin administration, participants were studied for 48 hours.

Residual radioactivity was determined by placing a gamma counter 50 mm from the injection site and the radioactivity counted for 5 minute intervals at 1, 2, 4, 6, 8, 12, 16, 20, 24, 36 and 48 hours after injection. During the first 24 hour period, patients remained fasted and samples were taken for blood glucose and C-peptide measurement.

The rate of absorption from subcutaneous tissue was calculated from levels of residual radioactivity following injection of [^{125}I]-labeled insulin. The primary pharmacokinetic endpoint was the time in hours for 25% of the administered radioactivity to disappear (T$_{75}$%). Secondary variables were the times taken for 50% and 75% of the administered radioactivity to disappear (T$_{50}$% and T$_{25}$%) and the mean residual radioactivity at the injection site 24, 36 and 48 hours after injection. The primary pharmacodynamic variables were plasma glucose and C-peptide concentrations.

KEY FINDINGS

- Median values for disappearance of radioactivity were significantly longer for insulin glargine compared with NPH insulin (Table 4).
- The median residual radioactivity at the injection site was significantly higher for insulin glargine compared to NPH insulin (Figure 30 and Table 5).
- Mean plasma glucose levels reached a minimum after 14.6 ± 1.3 hours and 9.0 ± 2.0 hours in response to insulin glargine and NPH insulin, respectively.

T$_{25}$%	=	15.0 vs. 6.5 hours,	p=0.009
T$_{50}$%	=	26.3 vs. 13.4 hours,	p=0.009
T$_{75}$%	=	42.4 vs. 26.6 hours,	p=0.019

Table 4. Residual radioactivity.

24 hours	=	54.4 vs. 27.9%,	p=0.0001
36 hours	=	35.0 vs. 17.0%,	p=0.003
48 hours	=	19.2 vs. 9.2%,	p=0.01

Table 5. Residual radioactivity.

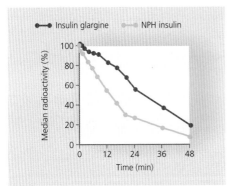

Figure 30. Disappearance of radiolabeled insulin over time after injection subcutaneous injection into the anterior abdominal wall. (Reprinted from *Hormone and Metabolic Research* 2003; 35:434–438. Reprinted with permission from the Thieme Publishing Group).

EDITORS COMMENTARY

This study demonstrated a much slower rate of disappearance of insulin glargine from subcutaneous tissue than NPH insulin in persons with T2DM.This finding is in keeping with an earlier study that documented a longer presence of glargine in subcutaneous tissue than NPH insulin in healthy subjects. This slow absorption profile of insulin glargine reduces the likelihood of peaks of action, which has obvious potential clinical applications.

Additional references

1. Luzio SD, Owens D, Evans M, Ogunku A, Beck P, Kurzhals R. Comparison of the sc absorption of HOE 901 and NPH human insulin type 2 diabetic subjects. *Diabetes* 1999; 48(Suppl 1):A111 Abstract 0480.

Abstract

Comparison of biphasic insulin aspart (BIAsp 30) and insulin glargine (IGlarg) during isoglycaemic clamp studies in persons with type 2 diabetes.

Luzio S, Peter R, Dunseath G, Pauvaday V, Owens DR. *Diabetes* 2004; 53:(Suppl 2)A136 Abstract 573-P.

Following injection of BIAsp 30 insulin, the plasma insulin concentrations increased rapidly, reaching distinct peaks 2 - 3 hours after injection, in contrast to insulin glargine which had a peakless profile with a plateau between 6 - 16 hours.

STUDY RATIONALE

In current clinical practice for persons with T2DM the next treatment step after treatment failure with OHAs is supplementation with insulin. This may be achieved by either the introduction of a basal insulin preparation with continued OHAs or a premixed insulin preparation which provides both basal and prandial insulin requirements. This study was undertaken to evaluate these two very different approaches to insulin therapy by comparing the pharmacokinetic and pharmacodynamic profiles of BIAsp 30 administered twice-daily and insulin glargine administered once-daily at the same total daily dose.

OBJECTIVES

To compare the pharmacokinetic and pharmacodynamic properties of BIAsp 30 and insulin glargine in persons with persons with T2DM.

SUBJECTS

Twelve persons with T2DM, insulin naïve and treated with diet and OHAs were enrolled (mean ± SD: age 58.8 ± 8.9 years, BMI 31.0 ± 3.0 kg/m² and HbA$_{1c}$ 7.1 ± 0.6 %).

STUDY DESIGN

In brief: A single-center, randomised, 24 hour isoglycemic clamp study comparing the effect of either 0.5 U/kg of BIAsp 30, given as two doses 12 hours apart (0.25 U/kg at 08:30 and 0.25 U/kg at 20:30) or the same total daily dose (0.5 U/kg) of insulin glargine at 08:30, both subcutaneously into the anterior abdominal wall.

This was a randomised, open, single-centre, two-way crossover study. Patients were studied on two separate study days, 7(±3) days apart. On study day one, subjects were randomised to receive either 0.5 U/kg of BIAsp 30 given as two doses 12 hours apart (0.25 U/kg at 08:30h and 0.25 U/kg at 20:30h) or the same total dose (0.5 U/kg) of insulin glargine at 08:30h both by subcutaneous (sc) administration into the anterior abdominal wall. An isoglycemic clamp was carried out over the following 24 hours. After a washout period of approximately 7 days, all 12 persons returned to the clinic for a further study day on which they received the comparator preparation.

During each of the study days, patients remained fasting and on bed rest during a 24 hour hypoglycemic "clamp" study. Fasting samples were taken at -30, -20, -10 and 0 minutes, following which a bolus dose of either 0.25 U/kg BIAsp 30 or 0.5 U/kg insulin glargine, according to a randomization schedule, was administered subcutaneously into a skin fold of the anterior abdominal wall.

Patients randomised to BIAsp 30 received a second dose (0.25 U/kg) 12 hours later. Samples for determination of plasma glucose concentrations were taken at 10-minute intervals. The glucose infusion rate was adjusted to maintain blood glucose concentrations at fasting levels. Frequent samples for plasma insulin and C-peptide concentrations were also taken over the 24-hour study period.

KEY FINDINGS

- The mean doses of BIAsp 30 (46.5 ± 5.6 U (range 36 - 50 U)) and insulin glargine (46.5 ± 5.4 U (range 37 – 50 U)) were comparable between treatment groups.
- Plasma glucose remained constant throughout the 24-hour clamp period. CV of plasma glucose during clamps (derived by calculating the CV of deviation (%) of all glucoses during the clamp from the target value) was 6.3% for BIAsp 30 and 4.3% for insulin glargine, respectively.
- Following each injection of BIAsp 30, GIR increased rapidly reaching a distinct peak (Figure 31). A flatter post-injection GIR profile was observed following injection of Insulin glargine.
- GIR AUC_{0-24h} was approximately 34% higher following BIAsp 30 than after insulin glargine (2.51 ± 0.36 vs. 1.87 ± 0.12 g/kg/minute, p=0.037).
- Plasma insulin rose more rapidly and had a higher peak following injection of BIAsp 30 than Insulin glargine. Insulin AUC_{0-24h} was 28.2% higher after BIAsp 30 than Insulin glargine (4514 ± 404 vs. 3521 ± 368 pmol/L/hour, p=0.001).
- Plasma C-peptide levels fell below baseline levels following both injections (A and B) of BIAsp 30 but were unchanged following injection of Insulin glargine.
- Over the 24-hour study period the C-peptide AUC_{0-24h} following BIAsp 30 was significantly lower than for insulin glargine (19.7 ± 2.4 vs. 22.4 ± 3.1 nmol/L/hour, p=0.029).

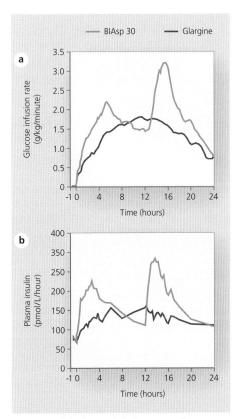

Figure 31. (**a**) Glucose infusion rates after subcutaneous injection. (**b**) Serum insulin concentrations after subcutaneous injection.

EDITOR'S COMMENTARY

This study shows that following each injection of BIAsp 30 insulin, plasma insulin concentrations increased rapidly reaching distinct peaks 2 - 3 hours after injection, in contrast to insulin glargine which had a peakless profile with a plateau between 6 - 16 hours. The glucose infusion rate reflected the insulin profiles. The AUC_{0-24h} for plasma insulin and GIR were approximately 30% higher following the two injections of BIAsp 30 than insulin glargine despite the same total daily dose.

Abstract

An assessment of the variability in the pharmacodynamics (glucose lowering effect) of HOE901 compared to NPH and ultralente human insulins using the euglycemic clamp technique.

Scholtz HE, Pretoruis SG, Wessels DH, Meyer BH, Van Niekerk N, Rosenkranz B. *Clinical Pharmacology and Therapeutics* 2000; 67(2):123 Abstract PII–36.

And

Reproducibility of serum insulin and glucose infusion rate profiles of insulin glargine compared with NPH insulin and insulin Ultralente.

Scholtz HE and Becker RHA. Diabetes 2004; 53(Suppl 2):Abstract 2011–PO.

The intra-subject coefficient of variability in glucose lowering effect with insulin glargine was comparable to NPH insulin and superior to ultralente insulin following subcutaneous administration. A re-analysis using non-parametric methods to account for poorly produced profiles in two subjects showed that insulin glargine is associated with 30 - 50% less day-to-day variability in GIR profile reproducibility compared to NPH insulin and Ultralente.

STUDY RATIONALE

NPH insulin and Ultralente insulin are characterized by poor reproducibility of serum insulin levels and in glucose lowering effect. Insulin glargine has a smooth, peakless time action profile, but the reproducibility of the glucose lowering response of insulin glargine was not defined.

OBJECTIVES

To compare the pharmacodynamic variability (glucose lowering effect) of subcutaneous insulin glargine, NPH insulin and Ultralente insulin in healthy volunteers using the "euglycemic" clamp technique.

STUDY DESIGN

A single dose, double-blind, randomized, parallel replicate "euglycemic" clamp study undertaken in healthy male subjects assessing between day and within-subject variations in serum insulin concentration and the corresponding glucose lowering effect.

In this double-blind, randomized, parallel replicate design study, 36 healthy male volunteers aged 18 – 45 years were enrolled in three treatment groups (n=12/group). Subjects received two consecutive subcutaneous injections of insulin glargine, NPH insulin or ultralente insulin (0.4 units/kg), with a wash-out period of 7 days between treatments. "Euglycemic" clamps were performed, for up to 24 hours, after subcutaneous administration of the insulins 'clamped' at the subjects' individual fasting blood glucose concentration.

The area under the curve (AUC) of the glucose infusion rate (GIR) (mg/kg) was the main pharmacodynamic variable and was recorded every 10 minutes for 24 hours. Insulin concentrations, corrected for endogenous insulin, were determined every hour.

In the first study, the mean values and coefficients of variation were determined for each of the patient groups. In the second analysis, the profile reproducibility and the standard deviation of these differences were calculated.

- The profile reproducibility was defined as the cumulative absolute differences in insulin concentration and GIR (clamp 1 - clamp 2) (ΔINS–CUM$_{absolute}$).
- The standard deviation of these differences was calculated to display a measure of the spread of these differences over time (SD–ΔINS$_{raw}$).

	Glargine/NPH	Glargine/Ultralente
Peak Exposure (90%CI)		
$INS-AUC_{0-24h}$	0.64 (0.53,0.77)	0.89 (0.74,1.08)
$GIR-AUC_{0-24h}$	0.93 (0.67,1.28)	1.20 (0.83,1.79)
Ratio (median)		
$\Delta INS-CUM_{absolute}$	0.52; 0.81**	0.32
$\Delta GIR-CUM_{absolute}$	0.94	0.60
$SD-\Delta INS_{raw}$	0.62; 0.94**	0.50
$SD-\Delta GIR_{raw}$	0.71	0.49
**normalized for $INS-AUC_{0-24h}$		

Table 6. Summary of principle findings.

The cumulative differences are similar to the area between the curves as the values were taken every 10 minutes for GIR and hourly for insulin. Non-parametric tests (Kruskal-Wallace) were employed.

KEY FINDINGS

- In the first analysis, intra-subject coefficient of variation during the 24 hour 'clamp' (AUC 12-24 hours) period (AUC 0-24 hours) was lowest for NPH insulin (19%) followed by insulin glargine (32%) and ultralente insulin (38%).
- Between 12 and 24 hours during the 'clamp' period, intra-subject variability was lowest for insulin glargine (23%) followed by NPH insulin (29%) and ultralente insulin (55%).
- In the second analysis, total insulin exposure ($INS-AUC_{0-24h}$) was 40% greater for NPH insulin compared to insulin glargine, but suppression of endogenous insulin release (C-peptide) and total glucose disposal ($GIR-AUC_{0-24h}$) were similar for all groups (Table 6).
- The profile reproducibility was the same for insulin glargine and NPH insulin, but

significantly larger for Ultralente (Table 6).
- The standard deviation of between day differences in insulin and GIR showed less variation for insulin glargine profiles as compared with NPH and ultralente. However, these did not reach statistical significance because two subjects treated with insulin glargine were identified with markedly different profiles in exposure and hence GIR (Table 6).

Additional references

1. Scholtz HE, van Niekerk N , Meyer BH, Rosenkranz B. An assessment of the variability in the pharmacodynamics (glucose lowering effect) of HOE901 compared to NPH and ultralente human insulins using the euglycaemic clamp technique. *Diabetologia* 1999; 42(Suppl 1):A234 Abstract 882.

EDITORS COMMENTARY

Determination of intra-subject variability with different insulins is a challenging task. The extrapolation of the findings to the clinical arena is confounded by the magnitude of the variability and multiple factors that determine blood glucose levels. This type of study conducted under rigorous experimental conditions allows correction for certain variables like proper resuspension of NPH insulin and Ultralente and does provide useful, but not definitive, evidence on reproducibility.

The findings were initially presented in 1999 and 2000 and confirmed that insulin glargine had a peakless onset of action after 2 -3 hours, which was sustained for more than 24 hours and was consistent between visits. In contrast, the GIR profile of ultralente showed marked differences between the 2 visits, with about a four hour difference in onset of action (about 3 hours and 7 hours after administration). The intra-subject variation was lowest for NPH insulin (19%) followed by insulin glargine (32%) and ultralente insulin (38%), but was lowest for insulin glargine in the 12-24 hour period after injection. It is important to note that with this sort of analysis, the presence of a consistent peak for NPH insulin favors its reproducibility assessment.

In the data, it was apparent that the insulin glargine profiles were particularly poorly reproduced in 2 subjects, for unknown reasons. The re-analysis of the study findings, undertaken using non-parametric methods to give the extreme findings less weight, shows that insulin glargine is associated with 30 - 50% less day-to-day variability in GIR profile reproducibility compared to NPH insulin and Ultralente.

Fluctuation of serum insulin levels after single and multiple dosing of insulin glargine.

Gerich J, Bolli G, Becker R, Zhu R. *Diabetologia* 2003; 46(Suppl 2):Abstract 783.

Insulin glargine exhibits less fluctuation in serum insulin levels compared to NPH insulin or ultralente.

STUDY RATIONALE

Of clinical concern are the large fluctuations of serum insulin concentrations in persons with DM treated with NPH insulin and ultralente. The within-day fluctuation of insulin glargine levels were undefined.

OBJECTIVES

To establish the level of fluctuation from mean serum levels of insulin glargine in comparison to other insulins using an analytical method, applied to previously described study findings.

STUDY DESIGN

Data from three previously described studies were assessed for fluctuations in mean serum insulin levels after single dose administration using analytical methods.

A complex fluctuation analysis tool, which was used to calculate fluctuation values based on the geometric mean values over a 24 hour period, expressed the findings as F_{24} alone and F_{24} as a percentage of average concentration (C_{ave}), expressed as PF_{24}. Three studies were analyzed that described findings in subjects with T1DM (2 studies, not described here) or healthy subjects (Scholtz et al., 1999). Healthy subjects (n=36) had received a single dose of insulin glargine, NPH insulin or ultralente (0.4 U/kg) on separate days (detailed on page 60).

KEY FINDINGS

In healthy subjects, pairwise comparisons of F_{24} showed significantly less fluctuation in mean serum insulin levels after a single dose of insulin glargine, in comparison to NPH insulin and to ultralente (Figure 32).

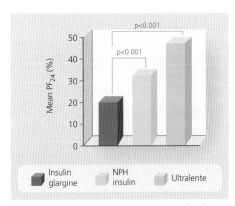

Figure 32. Fluctuation in serum insulin levels reported in Scholtz et al., 1999.

EDITORS COMMENTARY

Reviewing healthy subjects only, the analysis of within-day fluctuations of serum insulin levels shows that insulin glargine offers a more consistent serum level compared to NPH insulin and ultralente. This may potentially reduce episodes of hyperglycemia or hypoglycemia.

Abstract

24h profile of action of biosynthetic long-acting insulin (HOE901) tested in normal volunteers by glucose clamp methodology.

Soon PC, Matthews DR, Rosskamp R, Herz M, Kurzhals R. *Diabetes* 1997; 46(Suppl 1):161A Abstract 0621.

Insulin glargine has an extended plateau profile of action, offering suitability for overnight use as basal insulin.

STUDY RATIONALE

The insulin analog, insulin glargine, was known to have an extended duration of action, but required further study.

OBJECTIVES

To compare the 24 hour pharmacodynamic activity profile of insulin glargine compared to NPH and Ultratard insulins using the glucose clamp technique in healthy subjects following bolus subcutaneous administration.

STUDY DESIGN

Twelve healthy subjects were 'clamped' at a blood glucose concentration of 81 mg/dL (4.5 mmol/L) for 24 hours on separate occasions following subcutaneous injection of either insulin glargine, NPH insulin or Ultratard insulin.

Twelve healthy male subjects were studied for 24 hours on three separate occasions at least 10 days apart. On each study day, subjects received a bolus subcutaneous injection of insulin glargine, NPH insulin or Ultratard insulin at 6 PM. A variable rate intravenous glucose infusion was used to maintain blood glucose at 81 mg/dL (4.5 mmol/L) for the 24 hour study period.

KEY FINDINGS

- At 6 hours following subcutaneous insulin administration, the glucose infusion rate peaked at 1.4 mg/kg/minute for insulin glargine, 3.5 mg/kg/minute for NPH insulin and 0.8 mg/kg/minute for Ultratard insulin ($p<0.001$).
- At 14-16 hours following insulin administration, the glucose infusion rate was 2.5mg/kg/minute for all three insulins with no significant difference between profiles throughout the rest of the 24 hour study period.
- Exogenous serum insulin (calculated from the total insulin concentration corrected using the C peptide concentration) rose to 10 µU/ml at 5 hours for insulin glargine, 25 µU/ml at 4 hours for NPH insulin and 9 µU/ml at 14-22 hours for Ultratard insulin.
- Exogenous serum insulin remained at a plateau for insulin glargine.

EDITORS COMMENTARY

This small study, published only as an abstract, offers limited information, including no details of site of subcutaneous injection or dose of insulin. The results offer some confirmatory data on the pharmacodynamics of insulin glargine, showing an extended plateau profile compared to NPH insulin and Ultratard insulin, suggesting that insulin glargine has distinct basal insulin characteristics.

Physiological responses during hypoglycemia induced by regular human insulin or a novel human analog, insulin glargine.

Dagogo-Jack S, Askari H, Morrill B, Lehner LL, Kim B, Sha X. *Diabetes, Obesity and Metabolism* 2000; 2:373-383.

Insulin glargine is not associated with significant alterations in physiological or biochemical responses to hypoglycemia when compared to regular human insulin.

STUDY RATIONALE

Shortly after human insulin was introduced as a replacement for animal insulins, there were reports from patients of an altered perception of hypoglycemic symptoms. This study examined if the difference between insulin glargine and regular insulin translates into alterations in physiological response to hypoglycemia.

OBJECTIVES

To compare the physiological symptoms, and counter-regulatory hormones during hypoglycemia induced by regular human insulin or insulin glargine in healthy subjects and in persons with T1DM.

STUDY DESIGN

A single-dose, double-blind, randomized, two-way crossover trial in healthy subjects and persons with T1DM, assessing the nocturnal counter-regulatory response and a range of symptoms during a stepped hypoglycemic clamp using regular human insulin or insulin glargine.

Six healthy subjects and 13 persons with T1DM were enrolled in a single-dose, double-blind, randomized, two-way crossover trial. Subjects underwent a stepped hypoglycemic clamp procedure in which a continuous intravenous infusion of human insulin or insulin glargine was used to lower blood glucose levels in a series of 5 steps from 4.7 to 2.5 mmol/L. A simultaneous infusion of dextrose was used to maintain euglycemia. A symptom scoring system based on the intensity of neurogenic symptoms (sweating, heart pounding and palpitations, tremor, hunger, nervousness and tingling) and neuroglycopenic symptoms (difficulty in thinking, tiredness, dizzyness, weakness, and blurred vision) was used to assess perception of hypoglycemia. Plasma samples were taken at regular intervals to measure counter-regulatory hormones and substrates. The procedure was repeated with the comparative insulin after a 7-14 day washout period.

KEY FINDINGS

- Controlled hypoglycemia induced by intravenous infusions of human insulin and insulin glargine each produced a similar and significant increase in the total symptom score in normal individuals.
- The peak total symptom scores at the lowest blood glucose level (2.5 mmol/L) elicited by human insulin and insulin glargine were comparable in both normal subjects (human insulin: 18.83 ± 2.68; insulin glargine: 18.5 ± 3.20) and in persons with T1DM (human insulin: 17.46 ± 3.62; insulin glargine: 19.08 ± 3.83).
- The peak epinephrine levels in normal subjects during hypoglycemia induced by human insulin and insulin glargine were comparable (767 ± 140.4 pg/ml and and 608.8 ± 129.9 pg/ml respectively).
- Human insulin and insulin glargine elicited similar rates of glucose disposal.

Additional references

1. Dagogo Jack S, Askari H, Lehner LL. Effect of glargine on glucose disposal and lipolysis in healthy and diabetic subjects. *Diabetes* 2000; 49(Suppl 1) A412 Abstract 1737–PO.

2. Askari H, Lehner LL, Dagogo Jack S. Effects of insulin glargine, hypoglycaemia and counterregulation. *Diabetes* 2000; 49(Suppl 1):A411 Abstract 1735–PO.

EDITORS COMMENTARY

Symptoms were experienced in equivalent degrees during hypoglycemia induced by both insulins. The counter-regulatory hormone response did not differ significantly between the two insulins. Comparing human insulin and insulin glargine, the study found similar glucose infusion rates were required during the clamp procedure indicating that the insulins are equipotent with regard to a key biologic property, namely insulin-stimulated glucose disposal. These findings indicate that the structural and physicochemical properties of insulin glargine are not associated with significant alterations in physiological or biochemical responses to controlled hypoglycemia compared to regular human insulin in normal subjects and persons with T1DM. Thus, it is unlikely that insulin glargine has any intrinsic role in the genesis of hypoglycemia unawareness. Nevertheless, further studies to assess the responses to insulin glargine in subjects with previous evidence of hypoglycemia unawareness are certainly warranted.

Equipotency of insulin glargine and regular human insulin on glucose disposal in healthy subjects following intravenous infusion.

Scholtz HE, Pretorius SG, Wessels DH, Venter C, Potgieter MA, Becker RHA. Acta *Diabetologia* 2003; 40:156–162.

Equimolar concentrations of insulin glargine and regular insulin administered by intravenous infusion in healthy subjects have equivalent glucose lowering effects using a 6 hour "euglycemic" glucose clamp.

STUDY RATIONALE

The glucose lowering effect of insulin glargine in comparison with regular human insulin was investigated.

OBJECTIVES

To compare the glucose-lowering effect of equimolar concentrations of insulin glargine and regular semi-synthetic human soluble insulin given intravenously in healthy subjects using the 'euglycemic' clamp technique.

STUDY DESIGN

Twenty healthy subjects received insulin glargine and regular insulin as a constant intravenous infusion followed by a 'euglycemic' glucose clamp.

This study was a single dose, double-blind, randomized two-way crossover study in which healthy subjects (n=20) received insulin glargine and regular insulin (0.1 U/kg) as a 30 minute constant intravenous infusion after which they were clamped for six hours at their individual fasting blood glucose concentration. The area under the curve (AUC) of the glucose infusion rate (GIR) was calculated.

KEY FINDINGS

- The $AUC_{(0-6)}$ of the GIR for insulin glargine and regular insulin was 663.9 and 734.9 mg/kg, respectively.
- The 90% confidence interval for the mean ratio of insulin glargine to regular insulin

was 84.6 – 96.7% (point estimate 90.3%), which was within the pre-defined equivalence range.

EDITORS COMMENTARY

In healthy subjects equimolar concentrations of insulin glargine and regular insulin administered by short intravenous infusion have equivalent glucose lowering effects using the "euglycemic" glucose clamp technique over a six hour period. The intravenous route of administration of insulin glargine is not approved and is not the recommended route of administration. Nonetheless, the intravenous route was used in this study as a valid approach to assess the intrinsic potency of insulin glargine. This finding has some relevance to clinical practice. This study shows the possibility of rapid action of insulin glargine if the subcutaneous injection inadvertently hits a small blood vessel.

Additional References

1. Meyer BH, Sholtz HE, Pretorius SG, van Niekerk N, Rosenkranz B. A comparison of the pharmacodynamics (glucose lowering effect) of intravenous HOE901 and regular insulin using the euglycemic clamp technique. *Clinical Pharmacology and Therapeutics* 2000; 67(2):123 Abstract PII–34.

2. Meyer BH, Sholtz HE, Van Niekerk N, Rosenkranz B. A comparison of the pharmacodynamics (glucose lowering effect) of intravenous HOE901 and regular insulin using the euglycamic clamp technique. *Diabetologia* 1999; 42(Suppl 1):A234 Abstract 881.

Intravenous glargine and regular insulin have similar effects on endogenous glucose output and peripheral activation/deactivation kinetic profiles.

Mudaliar S, Mohideen P, Deutsch R, Ciaraldi TP, Armstrong D, Kim B, Sha X. Henry RR.

Diabetes Care 2002; 25:1597–602.

Although insulin glargine has an amino acid sequence distinct from human insulin, when given intravenously it has similar biological activity, as measured by hepatic glucose output and peripheral glucose uptake.

STUDY RATIONALE

Insulin glargine has an amino acid sequence distinct from that of human insulin, which results in kinetic differences. Absorption is delayed, but it was unclear if the amino acid changes alter biological activity.

OBJECTIVES

To compare the effects of intravenously administered insulin glargine and regular human insulin on the activation and deactivation of suppression of endogenous glucose output (EGO) and stimulation of peripheral glucose disposal in healthy subjects.

STUDY DESIGN

Single dose, double blind, randomized cross-over study in healthy subjects using euglycemic glucose "clamp" technique and [^{3}H]-glucose.

Healthy subjects (n=12, age 34.8 ± 2.7 years, BMI 24.2 ± 0.7 kg/m², mean fasting plasma glucose 89 ± 2.2 mg/dL (4.9 ± 0.1 mmol/L) mean fasting insulin 8.1 ±2.4 uU/ml) took part in the glucose "clamp" study, which consisted of a basal study period and a glucose clamp study period.

After an eight hour overnight fast, subjects were infused with [^{3}H]-glucose (0.15 µCi/min) for five hours from ~3.00 AM. Plasma glucose, specific glucose activity and plasma insulin, immediately prior to the start of the glucose clamp period, were measured.

After basal measurements were complete, a 10 minute priming dose was followed by a continuous intravenous infusion of 40 mU/m²/min for 4 hours of either insulin glargine or regular human insulin, followed by a 3-hour deactivation period. During the 7-hour period, subjects received a continuous, variable infusion of [^{3}H]-labeled glucose to maintain euglycemia at 90 mg/dL (5 mmol/L).

The glucose turnover rate was assessed during both basal and glucose clamp phases using the modified Steele equations for non-steady-state conditions.

In the basal state, EGO is equal to the rate of glucose appearance (R_a). During the insulin infusion and deactivation phases, EGO was calculated as the difference between the Ra and the infusion rate of exogenous glucose.

- A_{50}EGO is the time in minutes required for 50% of the active suppression of EGO after insulin infusion.

- D_{50}EGO is the time required to achieve 50% deactivation from maximum insulin induced suppression of EGO after cessation of insulin infusion.

- Incremental glucose disposal rate (IGDR) was defined as the difference between the basal glucose disposal rate (GDR) and GDR values during and after cessation of insulin infusion.

- A_{50}IGDR was defined as the time from basal glucose disappearance (R_d) to reach half maximum insulin-stimulated glucose disposal rate R_d.

- D_{50}IGDR was defined as the time required for deactivation from maximum insulin-stimulated GDR to half maximum GDR after cessation of insulin infusion.

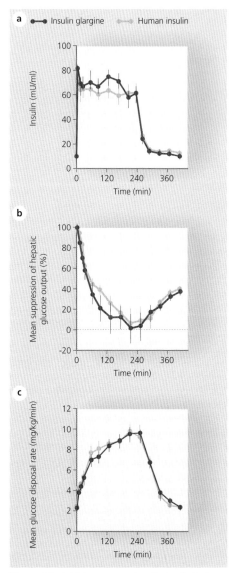

Figure 33. (**a**) Mean serum insulin levels during and after regular insulin and insulin glargine infusions. (**b**) Mean serum insulin levels during and after regular insulin and insulin glargine infusions. The results are means ± S.E. (**c**) Mean glucose disposal rates. The results are means ±S.E. ©2002 American Diabetes Association. *Diabetes Care* 2002; 25:1597–1602. Reprinted with permission.

KEY FINDINGS

No significant differences were observed in the activation and deactivation kinetics of intravenous administered insulin glargine and regular human insulin with respect to EGO or peripheral glucose disposal.

- Serum insulin concentrations of both were similar during the 4-hour insulin infusion (activation period) and during the 3-hour deactivation period (Figure 33a).
- The mean time required for 50% suppression of EGO ($A_{50}EGO$) after insulin infusion was similar for regular insulin (73 ± 23 minutes) and insulin glargine (57 ± 20 minutes) (Figure 33b).
- The mean maximum rate of glucose disposal was 10.10 ± 0.77 mg/kg/min for regular insulin and 9.90 ± 0.85 mg/kg/min for insulin glargine (Figure 33c).
- The mean time required for 50% suppression of the incremental GDR ($A_{50}IGDR$) was 32 ± 5 and 42 ± 10 minutes for regular insulin and insulin glargine respectively.
- The time required for deactivation from maximum insulin-stimulated GDR to half maximum GDR after cessation of insulin infusion ($D_{50}IGDR$) was 63 ± 5 and 57 ± 4 for regular insulin and insulin glargine respectively.

EDITORS COMMENTARY

These elegant findings show that insulin glargine does not differ from regular human insulin when administered intravenously in normal subjects. This provides good evidence that the different pharmacodynamic effects of regular insulin and insulin glargine observed following subcutaneous administration are due to differences in their absorption, with insulin glargine showing delayed absorption as a consequence of its distinct molecular structure.

Additional References

1. Mohideen P, Mudaliar S, Deutsch R, Ciaraldi TP, Armstrong D, Kim B, Morrill B. Characteristics of glucose turnover of insulin glargine in comparison with regular human insulin in healthy male subjects. *Diabetologia* 1999; 42(Suppl 1):A234 Abstract 879.

Biotransformation of insulin glargine after subcutaneous injection in healthy subjects.

Kuerzel GU, Shukla U, Scholtz HE, Pretorius S, Wessels DH, Venter C, Potgieter MA, Lang AM, Koose T, Bernhardt E. *Current Medical Research & Opinion* 2003; 19:34–40.

Insulin glargine undergoes metabolic breakdown both at the injection site and within the circulatory system to yield two products which are structurally similar to human insulin and which possess equivalent metabolic activity to the parent compound.

STUDY RATIONALE

In vivo animal studies have shown that two main metabolites of insulin glargine (designated M1 and M2) are produced. Metabolite one (M1) results from cleavage of the two arginine amino acids (B31 and B32) from the C terminus of the β chain (A21-Gly-insulin) and metabolite two (M2) from the additional loss of the next amino acid on the β chain (A21-Gly-des-30B-Thr-insulin). Both M1 and M2 have been shown to possess equivalent metabolic activity to that of the parent compound *in vitro* and *in vivo*.

OBJECTIVES

To determine the metabolic degradation pattern of insulin glargine in humans at the site of bolus subcutaneous injection and in the systemic circulation over 24 hours following administration.

STUDY DESIGN

Open label, metabolite-profiling study in five healthy subjects obtaining injection site tissue and plasma samples and using high performance liquid chromatography (HPLC) and radioimmunoassay (RIA) techniques to identify insulin glargine metabolites.

Five healthy, male subjects aged 18-50 years with a BMI of 18-26 kg/m^2 were enrolled. Four subjects received a single subcutaneous injection of insulin glargine (0.6 U/kg) into the anterior abdominal wall; placebo was administered to one subject. Subjects underwent a euglycemic glucose "clamp" procedure over the following 24 hour.

Blood samples were taken at one hour intervals and RIA was used to determine immunoreactive insulin (in plasma and serum) and C-peptide (in serum) concentrations. A tissue sample was obtained by liposuction from the point of subcutaneous injection. One tissue sample was taken at either 2, 6 12 or 24 hours after injection. Fractions containing insulin and insulin metabolites were identified by HPLC based on their retention times using reference compounds. The identity of insulin and insulin metabolites was confirmed by mass spectrometry.

KEY FINDINGS

- Analysis of tissue samples by HPLC and RIA revealed two immunoreactive peaks in varying ratios; the peak eluted first was identified as insulin glargine; the second peak was a mixture of metabolites, M1 and M2. Insulin glargine and the M1 and M2 metabolites were present in an average ratio of 50:50.
- Analysis of plasma samples revealed the presence of insulin glargine and two of the degradation products (M1 and M2) in the circulation in addition to endogenous insulin.

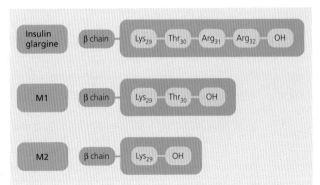

Figure 34. Endogenous insulin-like degradation.

EDITORS COMMENTARY

This study examined the 24 hour degradation profile of insulin glargine. Following subcutaneous administration, insulin glargine undergoes metabolic degradation resulting in two metabolites (M1 and M2). Degradation appears to be initiated at the injection site and continued within the circulatory system. The early degradation of insulin glargine in the subcutaneous tissue does not impair its biological activity.

Additional references

1. Kuerzel GU, Sandow J, Seipke G, Lang AM, Mass J, Skzipczyk HJ. Kinetics and Metabolite profile of insulin glargine (Lantus®). *Diabetologia* 2001; 44 (Suppl 1):A208 Abstract 798.

Metabolic action and cellular processing and degradation of insulin glargine.

Duckworth WC, Tsui BT, Fawcett J. *Diabetes Metabolism* 2003; 29(Spec No 2):Abstract 1656.

Certain differences in cellular processing and metabolic action occur between regular insulin and insulin glargine

STUDY RATIONALE

The effects of insulin glargine on glucose metabolism and mitogenesis have been extensively investigated as part of its safety evaluation, but other aspects of insulin glargine cellular processing and action have been studied in less detail.

OBJECTIVES

To compare insulin glargine to human insulin using HepG2 and 3T3-L1 cell line models to characterize cellular binding, degradation, intracellular processing, and stimulation of DNA synthesis. To study the relative impact of human insulin and insulin glargine on insulin-mediated lipolysis and glucose incorporation into lipids.

STUDY DESIGN

[^{125}I]-radiolabeled regular human insulin and insulin glargine were used to assess their respective cellular binding, degradation, intracellular processing, mitogenic potency (assessed by thymidine incorporation) and inhibition of epinephrine-stimulated lipolysis in HepG2 cells and 3T3-L1 cell lines.

In HepG2 cells, the cellular binding, degradation and processing of [^{125}I]-labeled human insulin and [^{125}I]-labeled insulin glargine were

quantified and effects on DNA synthesis (assessed by thymidine uptake) and protein degradation were measured. The effects of human insulin and insulin glargine on epinephrine-stimulated lipolysis and glucose incorporation into lipids were studied in 3T3-L1 adipocytes.

KEY FINDINGS

- The cellular binding of human insulin and insulin glargine were similar in HepG2 cells.
- Degradation of human insulin was significantly higher than insulin glargine (21.6 ± 1.4% vs. 16.3 ± 0.3% degraded/hour; p<0.01) and consequently more degraded human insulin was released, by cells previously loaded with radiolabeled material, compared to insulin glargine (58.3 ± 1.4% vs. 50.1 ± 2.4%; p<0.02). The amount of intact human insulin was concomitantly reduced compared with insulin glargine (35.8 ± 1.4% vs. 44.8 ± 2.6%; p<0.02).
- Protein degradation was significantly higher (~20%) with human insulin compared to insulin glargine (~15%; p<0.05).
- In 3T3-L1 adipocytes, human insulin inhibited epinephrine-stimulated lipolysis to a greater degree compared to insulin glargine (EC$_{50}$= 0.35 vs. 1.40 nM; p<0.001).
- Human insulin and insulin glargine had similar effects on lipogenesis and glucose oxidation to CO$_2$.

EDITORS COMMENTARY

The assessment of insulin analogs and how their metabolic processing, binding and actions compares to human insulin have not been extensively investigated. Previous studies have however suggested that the mechanism of insulin action is not exclusively related to the extent of receptor-binding and receptor-mediated signal transduction. This study demonstrates *in vitro* differences in metabolic action and cellular processing between regular human insulin and intact insulin glargine in the cell lines studied. Intracellular processing and degradation of insulin glargine was less than human insulin and more intact insulin glargine was released by cells compared with regular insulin. Insulin glargine was also slightly less effective in reducing lipolysis and inhibiting protein degradation. However, these differences are considered unlikely to have adverse clinical effects and may even partially enhance the effectiveness of insulin glargine as a basal insulin.

Abstract

Effects of basal insulin treatment on IGF-1: glargine vs. NPH-insulin.

Slawik M, Petersen KG. *Diabetes* 2002; 51(Suppl 1):A296 Abstract 1202–P.

Insulin glargine has no intrinsic *in vivo* IGF-1 affinity.

STUDY RATIONALE

Given the role of the IGF-1 receptor in mediating aberrant insulin growth signals and the 6-8 fold higher affinity of insulin glargine for the IGF-1 receptor shown in a specific *in vitro* model, *in vivo* assessments of the effect of insulin glargine on IGF-1 levels were warranted.

OBJECTIVES

To determine if insulin glargine has intrinsic IGF-1 activity *in vivo*, determined indirectly by assessing serum IGF-1 levels in comparison to NPH insulin in persons with T1DM and T2DM.

STUDY DESIGN

Single center, open label study measuring IGF-1 concentrations in serum, one and three weeks after commencement of treatment with either insulin glargine or NPH insulin.

Subjects with T1DM (n=15; mean age: 27 years; mean BMI: 25 kg/m²) or T2DM (n=20; mean age: 66 years; mean BMI: 30 kg/m²) being treated with either NPH insulin or insulin glargine, were switched to the alternative insulin for 3 weeks. Serum IGF-1 and HbA_{1c} were measured at one and three weeks.

KEY FINDINGS

• No reduction in serum IGF-1 values was detected in response to insulin glargine compared to NPH insulin (Figure 35) in persons with T1DM or T2DM.

• The serum IGF-1 levels increased moderately with insulin glargine and this was most marked in males with T1DM.

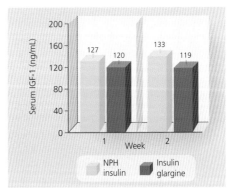

Figure 35. Serum IGF-1 concentrations in combined group of patients with T1DM or T2DM.

EDITORS COMMENTARY

The measurement of IGF-1 levels was an indirect means of examining the interaction of NPH insulin and insulin glargine with the IGF-1 receptor. Since IGF-1 levels did not decrease when patients were switched from NPH to insulin glargine, no intrinsic binding activity of insulin glargine at the IGF-1 receptor *in vivo* is suspected.

Vascular function; retinopathy

Progression of retinopathy with insulin glargine or NPH insulin: A multi-trial analysis.

Abstract

Forjanic-Klapproth J, Home PD. *Diabetologia* 2001; 44(Suppl 1):A287 Abstract 1103.

This comprehensive analysis of data from four phase III clinical trials in persons with T1DM and T2DM was conducted by an expert panel and provides strong evidence and opinion that insulin glargine is not associated with an increased risk of, or progression of, diabetic retinopathy.

STUDY RATIONALE

Given the awareness of the role of the IGF-1 receptor in mediating aberrant insulin growth signals and the implication of IGF-1 as a mediator of progression of retinopathy, an expert panel was convened and a detailed review conducted of four phase III registration studies. The panel sought evidence that there was no association between insulin glargine therapy and diabetic retinopathy progression.

OBJECTIVES

To examine in detail the adverse opthalmological outcomes in persons with T1DM or T2DM who had been treated with insulin glargine or NPH insulin within a defined clinical trial environment.

STUDY DESIGN

Retrospective assessment of parameters related to ophthalmologic safety in persons with T1DM or T2DM enrolled in four randomized clinical trials.

The findings of the comprehensive ophthalmologic-related safety parameters included in the four phase III randomized clinical trials in 2207 persons with T1DM or T2DM were reviewed by an expert panel, consisting of four ophthalmologists and one physician, considered experts in the field.

The assessments reviewed were:
- Progression of retinopathy (≥3 steps of the ETDRS)
- Development of proliferative retinopathy (ETDRS ≥61)
- Clinically significant macular edema (CSME)
- Retinal Adverse Events (RAES)
- Disc swelling

The examinations reviewed were:
- Ophthalmologic examination
- Fundus photography

KEY FINDINGS

- The rates of progression of retinopathy were shown to be similar between NPH insulin and insulin glargine, with the largest difference in a T2DM study (2.7% vs. 7.5%, respectively).
- Proliferative retinopathy rates appeared similar between NPH insulin and insulin glargine.
- The rates of CSME were not significantly different between NPH insulin and insulin glargine, based on ophthalmologic examination and fundus photography.
- A similar number of RAES (around 10%) were recorded with each treatment.
- Optic disc swelling was not observed in any patients.

	T1DM (n=1119)				T2DM (n=1088)			
	Pieber et al., 2000		Ratner et al., 2000		Yki-Järvinen et al., 2000		Rosenstock et al., 2001	
Finding	Insulin glargine	NPH insulin	Insulin glargine	NPH insulin	Insulin glargine	NPH insulin	Insulin glargine	NPH insulin
Progression of retinopathy								
Clinical exam	4.8	5.7	9.5	7.1	8.4	13.0	9.2	10.7
Photography	5.3	3.4	3.2	3.9	5.9	9.1	7.5	2.7
Proliferative retinopathy								
Clinical exam	1.9	1.1	1.3	1.7	0.7	0	2.7	1.3
Photography	2.2	2.6	1.8	3.8	2.1	1.8	4.1	2.2
New CSME								
Clinical exam	3.7	1.9	0.9	1.3	1.8	2.4	3.1	3.0
Photography	6.9	7.9	0.9	1.3	11.2	6.5	2.8	2.2
RAES	18.0	12.0	9.8	10.4	3.1	2.5	22.0	24.7
Disc swelling	0	0	0	0	0	0	0	0

EDITORS COMMENTARY

An extensive clinical evidence base (>2000 patients) from the registration trials was reviewed by the "Retinopathy Expert Working Group", an independent panel of four ophthalmologists and one endocrinologist, all with a special interest in diabetes. Their final conclusion, that "insulin glargine is not associated with increased risk of development or progression of diabetic retinopathy", appears to be valid from the detailed review that was undertaken.

There is an ongoing follow-up process, including data from clinical trial experience and post-marketing surveillance, to rule out any potential retinopathy-related long term effects of insulin glargine therapy.

3.5 years of insulin therapy with insulin glargine markedly improves *in vivo* endothelial function in type 2 diabetes.

Vehkavaara S, Yki-Järvinen H. *Arteriosclerosis, Thrombosis and Vascular Biology* 2004; 24:325–330.

Long-term insulin glargine markedly improved endothelium-dependent and endothelium-independent vasodilation in persons with T2DM.

STUDY RATIONALE

Endothelial dysfunction is an important finding in T2DM. Previous studies have shown that six months of insulin therapy with NPH insulin enhances both endothelium independent and dependent vasodilation in T2DM. The effects of prolonged insulin therapy with the insulin analog, insulin glargine, on vascular function are unknown.

OBJECTIVES

To determine whether long term insulin glargine therapy (3-5 years) maintains or further improves endothelial function in insulin-naïve patients with T2DM.

STUDY DESIGN

Comparison of endothelial function before and after the introduction of insulin glargine in persons with T2DM matched to healthy subjects. The endothelial function was estimated from blood flow response to *in vivo* intrabrachial artery infusions of endothelial dependent and independent vasodilators.

Subjects

Eleven insulin-naïve persons with T2DM receiving OHA (age 59 ± 2 years; BMI 29.7 ± 0.9 kg/m²; known duration of diabetes 8 ± 1 years) and 16 healthy, age, gender and weight-matched control subjects were enrolled.

Treatment groups

Participants with T2DM received a single subcutaneous injection of insulin glargine once daily at bedtime for 3.5 years with OHA continued unchanged. Control subjects received no treatment.

Methodology

In vivo endothelial function was evaluated from blood flow responses to intra-brachial artery infusions of endothelial-dependent (acetylcholine (ACh): doses 7.5 and 15 µg/min) and endothelial-independent (sodium nitroprusside (SNP): doses 3 and 10 µg/min) vasodilators before and after 0.5 and 3.5 years of insulin glargine treatment. BMI, insulin dose and glycemic control were measured at baseline, and after 6 months and 3.5 years.

KEY FINDINGS

- Before insulin glargine treatment, as expected the blood flow response to ACh was significantly lower in persons with T2DM compared with healthy controls (p=0.021), but not in response to SNP.
- After 6 months of insulin glargine treatment, blood flow responses to both ACh and SNP increased significantly and were no longer different from control (Figure 36a).
- After 3.5 years of insulin glargine treatment, blood flow during infusion of high dose ACh increased significantly from 8.8 ± 0.9 ml/dL per minute at baseline to 13.0 ± 1.9 ml/dL per minute at 6 months (p<0.05) and to 14.7 ± 1.6 ml/dL per minute at 3.5 years (p<0.01 vs. baseline) (Figure 36b).

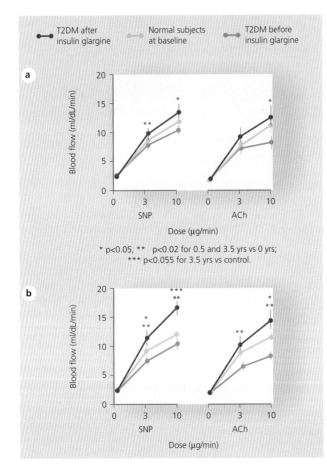

Figure 36. Forearm blood flow response to intra-arterial SNP and Ach infusions in (**a**) patients with T2DM at 6 months and (**b**) 3.5 years. (Reprinted from *Arteriosclerosis, Thrombosis and Vascular Biology* 2004; 24:1–7. Reprinted with permission from LWW Publishing Group).

- After 3.5 years of insulin glargine treatment, blood flow during infusion of SNP increased significantly from 10.7 ± 0.9 ml/dL per minute at baseline to 13.4 ± 1.0 ml/dL per minute at 6 months (p<0.01) and 16.6 ± 1.5 ml/dL per minute at 3.5 years (p<0.01 vs. 0 years) (Figure 36b).
- During insulin glargine therapy, mean HbA_{1c} levels decreased from $9.1 \pm 0.4\%$ to $7.5 \pm 0.2\%$ at 6 months (p<0.001) and remained at this level ($7.5 \pm 0.2\%$) at 3.5 years (p<0.001).
- The bedtime insulin glargine dose averaged 40 ± 5 IU (0.43 U/kg) at 6 months increasing to 60 ± 10 U (0.63 U/kg) at 3.5 years, there was no significant change in body weight during the study (87.5 ± 3.4, 88.7 ± 3.8 and 89.9 ± 3.9 kg at baseline, 6 months and 3.5 years, respectively).

EDITORS COMMENTARY

The effects of hyperinsulinemia on vascular function are continually debated. However, studies show that insulin therapy acutely enhances vasodilation induced by endothelium-dependent vasodilators, such as Ach and activates endothelial nitric oxide synthase increasing the production of nitric oxide *in vitro*.

A marked improvement in both endothelium-dependent and endothelium-independent vasodilation was seen at 6 months and a further improvement at 3.5 years from study initiation with insulin glargine treatment. These data support the view that insulin glargine therapy can improve and even reverse endothelial dysfunction and has reaffirmed the fact that insulin has beneficial rather than harmful effects on vascular function.

Additional references

1. Vehkavaara S, Yki-Järvinen H. 3.5 years of insulin therapy with insulin glargine at bedtime markedly improves *in vivo* endothelial function in type 2 diabetes. *Diabetes* 2002; 51(Suppl 2):A173 Abstract 699-P.

Glargine and regular human insulin similarly acutely enhance endothelium-dependent vasodilation in normal subjects

Westerbacka JJ, Bergholm R, Tiikainen M, Yki-Järvinen H. *Arteriosclerosis Thrombosis and Vascular Biology* 2004; 24:320–324

Insulin glargine and regular human insulin enhance the vasodilatory effect of acetylcholine to similar extents.

STUDY RATIONALE

The structural changes to insulin glargine may change its binding properties to the insulin receptor and homologous receptors, such as the insulin-like growth factor-1 receptor. Therefore, this study was carried out to examine the impact of insulin glargine on vascular function in normal subjects given that its *in vivo* effects on endothelium-dependent and endothelium-independent vascular function were previously unknown.

OBJECTIVES

To compare the *in vivo* effects in healthy subjects of regular human insulin and insulin glargine on endothelium-dependent and endothelium-independent vasodilation induced by acetyl choline (ACh) and sodium nitroprusside (SNP).

STUDY DESIGN

Normal subjects received infusions of ACh or SNP and blood flow responses were recorded by venous occlusion plethysmography under both normal and hyperinsulinemic conditions, using infusions of saline, regular human insulin or insulin glargine.

Normal, apparently healthy males (n=10; mean ± SD: age: 33 ± 3 years, mean BMI: 23.2 ± 2.4 kg/m^2) were studied on two days in a double-blind, cross-over fashion. Subjects were studied under normoglycemic or normoglycemic hyperinsulinemic "clamp" conditions maintained by intravenous infusion of saline, regular human insulin or insulin glargine (120 min, 1 mU/kg/min). In each study, blood flow responses to intrabrachial artery infusions of ACh and SNP were recorded.

KEY FINDINGS

- Comparing saline to insulin, endothelium-independent blood flow responses to low (3 µg/min) and high (10 µg/min) doses of SNP were unaltered by regular human insulin (11.2 ± 1.1 vs. 12.0 ± 1.7 and 16.8 ± 1.9 vs. 18.4 ± 2.6 ml/dL/min, respectively) or by insulin glargine (12.2 ± 2.6 vs.13.4 ± 4.6 and 19.1 ± 4.2 vs.19.6 ± 5.1 ml/dL/min, respectively), but with no difference evident between the insulins.

- Comparing saline to insulin, endothelium-dependent blood flow responses to both low (7.5 µg/min) and high doses (15 µg/min) of ACh were enhanced significantly by regular human insulin (at low dose 11.5 ± 6.0 vs. 15.8 ± 8.0 ml/dL/min, respectively ($p < 0.05$) and at high dose 14.0 ± 7.5 vs. 21.1 ± 10.4 ml/dL/min, respectively ($p < 0.01$)) and insulin glargine (at low dose 13.9 ± 4.8 vs. 19.3 ± 6.5 ml/dL/min, respectively ($p < 0.02$) and at high dose 17.3 ± 2.1 vs. 23.2 ± 3.1 ml/dL/min, respectively ($p < 0.02$)) but with no difference evident between the insulins.

EDITORS COMMENTARY

This study shows a similar acute stimulatory effect on endothelium-dependent vasodilation in normal individuals mediated by regular human insulin and insulin glargine. These results suggest that the difference in structure between insulin glargine and human insulin has no effect on the acute vasodilatory effect of Ach or SNP in a dose response study. These findings are important to consider in the context of an increased binding affinity of insulin glargine *in vitro* to the IGF-1 receptor and suggest that *in vivo*, the enhanced binding affinity has no differential effect on vasodilatory function with human insulin and insulin glargine behaving similarly in normal subjects.

Additional references

1. Westerbacka JJ, Bergholm R, Tiikainen M, Yki-Järvinen H. Glargine and regular human insulin similarly acutely enhance endothelium-dependent vasodilation in normal subjects. *Diabetes Metabolism* 2003; 29(Spec No 2):Abstract 1203.

SUMMARY

Developed by Aventis, insulin glargine is the first clinically available recombinant, long-acting insulin analog. The pharmacokinetic imperfections of conventional "intermediate" and "long-acting" insulin preparations used over the last 50 years limit their ability to simulate basal insulin secretion, a prerequisite to normalize glycemia. The occurrence of peak insulin concentrations resulting from their subcutaneous administration causes both an increased risk of hypoglycemia and, due to the limited and variable duration of action, hyperglycemia. The power of recombinant DNA technology to create the designer insulin, insulin glargine, with protracted action, which is administered as a solution without the need for resuspension represents a landmark in modern molecular medicine. A large pre-clinical and clinical investigation program has characterized the binding and signaling characteristics, mitogenic capacity, absorption, metabolism and time-action profile of insulin glargine, validating the molecular design of this molecule, and indicating that this novel insulin molecule provides a long-acting and peakless basal insulin supply.

MOLECULAR CHEMISTRY

Insulin glargine was developed on the novel premise that the introduction of amino acid modifications that increase the isoelectric point of the native insulin molecule towards neutrality would result in precipitation of the insulin in the subcutaneous compartment and result in delayed absorption. The first extended-action insulin analog made by this method was NovoSol Basal (GlyA21, ArgB27, ThrB30-NH2-insulin), which had an extremely protracted absorption. However, the development was discontinued due to reduced bioavailability (Jorgensen et al., 1989). On the basis of the same concept, a new and novel di-arginyl insulin analog was developed, but this was shown to have a shorter glucose-lowering action than NPH insulin (Zeuzem et al., 1990). It was after further research that an

additional modification, substituting a glycine residue at position A21, was shown to alter the kinetics, resulting in an extended duration of action.

The molecular consequences of these alterations made to native human insulin to create insulin glargine result in key advantages for the analog over conventional insulin preparations. The alteration of the isoelectric point renders the insulin glargine molecule insoluble at physiologic pH, which results in amorphous precipitation in the subcutaneous tissue and a slow, peakless release with extended action up to 24 hours. In addition, the solubility of insulin glargine at an acidic pH ensures that the molecule is in solution at the time of injection, removing all concerns over variability in dosing because of a lack of resuspension.

RECEPTOR BINDING, SIGNALING AND MITOGENICITY

The findings from the studies conducted on the rapid-acting insulin analog, Asp [B10], emphasize why close assessment of receptor binding, receptor signaling and mitogenic potential of insulin analogs must be a central goal. Insulin receptor affinity and metabolic potency of insulin molecules are known to correlate with mitogenic potential, and that this is also related to insulin receptor occupancy time and to IGF-1 receptor affinity, as shown with Asp [B10] (Berti et al., 1998). Amino acid substitutions can modify the tertiary structure of the insulin protein in a way that alters interaction with the insulin and IGF-1 receptors and potentially lead to modifications in downstream, intracellular insulin signaling patterns.

In the studies using rat-1 fibroblasts overexpressing the human insulin receptor, insulin glargine behaved in a similar manner to normal human insulin with respect to insulin receptor association/dissociation and phosphorylation/dephosphorylation of the receptor and known substrates in the intracellular signaling cascade (Berti et al., 1998). Both insulins produced similar growth promoting activity as shown by comparable levels of thymidine incorporation. These findings suggest that insulin glargine does not differ significantly from native human insulin with respect to its effects on early intracellular signaling and mitogenic potency.

The growth-promoting activities of insulin glargine and native human insulin mediated by the IGF-1 receptor were compared in muscle tissue using cardiac myoblasts (H9c2 cardiac myoblasts) as a cell model, which express high levels of IGF-1 receptors with no detectable insulin receptors (Bähr et al., 1997). The growth-promoting activities of insulin glargine and human insulin were essentially identical, despite a slightly higher affinity of insulin glargine for the IGF-1 receptor. This finding relates only to the interaction of insulin glargine with the IGF-1 receptor.

In contrast with the findings described above, a further study did find that insulin glargine had a 6.5-fold increased affinity for the IGF-I receptor protein purified from transfected Baby Hamster Kidney cells and an 8-fold increased mitogenic potency, assessed by [3H]-thymidine incorporation, compared with native insulin in human malignant osteosarcoma cell line Saos/B10 that predominantly expresses IGF-1 receptors (Kurzhals, 2000). These findings were reviewed in depth and expert opinion indicated that differences in the findings reported related to the unique characteristics of the cell models used, in particular differences in the relative expression of insulin and IGF-I receptors (Kellerer and Häring, 2001).

Recently, more studies conducted using human micro- and macrovascular endothelial cells that abundantly express IGF-1 receptors have been published. Again, although a difference in binding between human insulin and insulin glargine was apparent, this was only at very high concentrations (Chisalita and Arnqvist, 2004). A recent study has examined the interaction of insulin glargine with the IGF-1 receptor in vitro and in vivo. Using a sophisticated surface plasmon resonance

Biacore analysis, which monitors the progress of biomolecular interactions in real time, insulin glargine had about an 8-fold higher affinity for soluble IGF-1 receptor compared to human insulin, but a 10-fold lower affinity than IGF-I. In addition, insulin glargine had a 14-fold faster association-rate and an almost 2-fold faster dissociation-rate as compared with insulin (Ekström et al., 2004). An in vivo study was then undertaken in 12 adolescents with T1DM who were about to receive a 12-week intensified treatment program with insulin glargine. IGF-I concentrations increased markedly after 2 weeks of insulin glargine treatment to a level sustained to study end. The authors suggest that this study confirms that insulin glargine has increased affinity for soluble IGF-1 receptor in vitro but that the increase in serum IGF-I concentrations argues against insulin glargine interactions with IGF-1 receptor in subjects with T1DM.

The findings that insulin glargine does have a greater capacity to promote DNA synthesis in certain situations compared to human insulin raised concerns, especially given that IGF-1 signaling is known to promote vascular endothelial growth factor-dependant retinal neovascularization, shown in Figure 37. Given this, an independent panel of experts retrospectively reviewed clinical data from 2207 patients enrolled in the registration trials for insulin glargine in persons with T1DM and T2DM (Forjanic-Klapproth and Home, 2001). There was no overall independent increased risk of development or progression of retinopathy and no cases of optic disk swelling were reported with either insulin glargine or NPH insulin, which makes it highly unlikely to be a real concern.

Further carcinogenicity studies carried out on mice and rats show no neoplastic changes after treatment with human insulin or insulin glargine up to 12.5 U/kg/day in rats and mice up to 2-years (Stammberger et al., 2002) and there is no suggestion in Wistar rats and Himalayan rabbits that insulin glargine has reproductive toxicity or embryotoxicity.

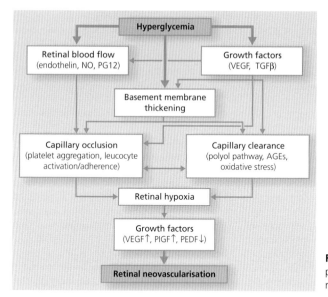

Figure 37. A model of the pathogenesis of diabetic retinopathy.

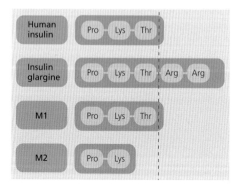

Figure 38. Metabolism of insulin glargine.

TIME ACTION PROFILES

The glucose-lowering effect of insulin glargine has been characterized using euglycemic glucose "clamp" studies. This technique determines insulin potency by measuring the continuous intravenous infusion of glucose needed to maintain euglycemia. In healthy subjects (Dreyer et al., 1994 and Heineman et al., 2000) or T1DM patients (Lepore et al., 2000 and Porcelatti et al., 2002) subcutaneous insulin glargine was shown to have a slower action onset, a prolonged duration of effect, and a relatively constant, flat time-action profile, compared to other insulins.

The early findings reported by Dreyer showed that insulin glargine was characterized by a longer duration of action with a less pronounced peak of insulin action compared to NPH insulin, irrespective of the zinc content of the formulation (Dreyer et al., 1994). The duration of insulin action was longer than 24 hours for both formulations of insulin glargine compared to NPH insulin, which had duration of action of about 16 hours.

The time-action profile of insulin glargine was described in comparison to NPH insulin over an extended period of 30 hours in healthy subjects using the "clamp" technique (Heinemann et al., 2000). The use of healthy subjects required endogenous insulin secretion to be suppressed, which was achieved by a continuous intravenous infusion of insulin. To correct for the metabolic effect of the infused insulin, a control experiment was conducted in which subjects received a placebo injection. Following subcutaneous injection, insulin glargine levels increased to a plateau within 4 hours of administration and remained constant thereafter, with no peak effect and almost constant glucose-lowering activity. The effect lasted up to an average of 24 hours, although in some patients the duration of action was estimated to be in excess of 30 hours (Heinemann et al., 2000).

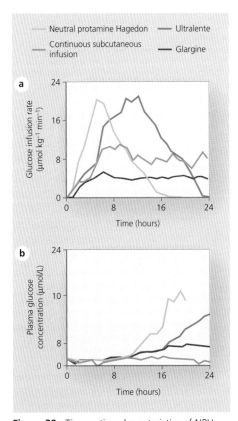

Figure 39. Time-action characteristics of NPH, Ultralente, glargine and continuous subcutaneous infusion with insulin lispro. The insulins were given by bolus subcutaneous injection in the medial aspect of the thigh at 0·3 U/kg, continuous subcutaneous infusion at 0·3 U/kg at time 0. (**a**) Glucose infusion rates to maintain plasma glucose at 7·2 mmol/L. (**b**) Corresponding plasma glucose concentrations. Intravenous glucose was withdrawn when glucose exceeded 7·5mmol. ©2000 American Diabetes Association. *Diabetes* 2000; 49:2142–2148. Reprinted with permission.

The results obtained in healthy subjects have been confirmed in intensively treated persons with T1DM. In a study undertaken in 20 subjects with T1DM to indirectly compare the pharmacokinetics and dynamics of insulin glargine with NPH insulin, ultralente and continuous subcutaneous infusion of insulin lispro (CSII), patients were studied on four occasions during a 24-hour isoglycemic clamp (Lepore et al., 2000). In a 2-way, crossover design patients were given 0.3 U/kg of insulin, either NPH insulin or insulin glargine subcutaneously. On two subsequent days, patients received either ultralente or CSII. There was a pronounced peak in action of human NPH insulin after about 4.5 hours and at about 10 hours after ultralente. Insulin glargine had a flat, prolonged action profile, with an onset of action was later than all other insulins (p<0.05) (Figures 39a and 39b). Additionally, intersubject variability was lower with insulin glargine than with human NPH insulin and ultralente (p<0.05).

In a comparison study (Porcellati et al., 2002), once daily insulin glargine given in the evening was compared to multiple daily injections of NPH insulin and continuous subcutaneous insulin infusion (CSII). The plasma glucose and insulin concentrations show that, compared to NPH insulin, insulin glargine and CSII provided less variable plasma glucose levels, without the glucose dip evident four hours after NPH administration. Plasma insulin levels were steady throughout the night, in contrast to the marked peak and trough associated with NPH insulin (Figure 40).

No differences between insulin glargine and NPH insulin in their ability to suppress endogenous hepatic glucose output during activation and deactivation periods or in the maximum rate of glucose disposal of the two types of insulin are described (Mudaliar, 2002), indicating that the different biological effects of insulin glargine and regular insulin observed following subcutaneous administration result from their different absorption kinetics.

The extended duration of action of insulin glargine does not lead to an accumulation of circulating insulin or an increased metabolic effect. Investigations in persons with T1DM

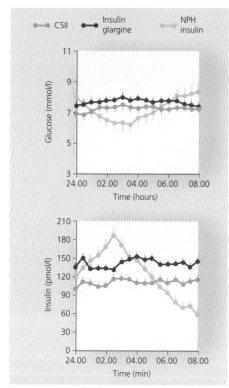

Figure 40. Nite-time plasma glucose and insulin levels after subcutaneous administration. Figure used with permission of Dr. F. Porcellati, MD, Perugia, Italy.

who received a single daily injection of insulin glargine at bedtime for 11 consecutive days show no accumulation following multiple injections over a 12 day dosing period and that the use of a loading dose or dose reduction after several injections of insulin glargine is unnecessary.

CONCLUSION

The insulin analog, insulin glargine, has a unique molecular structure, the biological consequences of which render the molecule long-acting with a predictable time-action profile and little intra-individual variability in bioavailability, and with no abnormal behavior with respect to mitogenicity.

References

1. Chisalita SI, Arnqvist HJ. Insulin-like growth factor 1 receptors are more abundant than insulin receptors in human micro- and macrovascular endothelial cells. *Am J Physiol Endocrinol Metab* 2004;286:E896-901.

2. Ekström K, Carlsson-Skwirut C, Salemyr J, Örtqvist E, Zachrisson I, Bang P. Evidence for interaction of insulin glargine with the type 1 IGF-1 receptor in vitro but not in vivo. *Diabetes* 2004; 53(Suppl 2): Abstract 523–P.

3. Jorgensen S, Vaag A, Langkjaer L, Hougaard P, Markussen J. Novo/Sol Basal: pharmacokinetics of a novel soluble long-acting soluble insulin analogue. *BMJ* 1989; 299:415–419.

4. Lepore M, Pampanelli S, Fanelli C, Porcellati F, Bartocci L, Di Vincenzo A, Cordoni C, Costa E, Brunetti P, Bolli GB. Pharmacokinetics and pharmacodynamics of subcutaneous injection of long-acting human insulin analog glargine, NPH insulin, and ultralente human insulin and continuous subcutaneous infusion of insulin lispro. *Diabetes* 2000: 49:2142–2148.

5. Owens DR, Zinman B, Bolli GB. Insulins today and beyond. *Lancet* 2001; 358:739–746.

6. Porcellati F, Pampanelli S, Fanelli C, Rosetti P, Torlone E, Costa E, Cordoni C, Brunetti P, Bolli GB. Comparison between different regimens of basal insulin supplementation in the prevention of nocturnal hypoglycemia in intensive treatment of Type 1 diabetes. *Diabetologia* 2001; 44(Suppl 1):Abstract 799.

7. Zeuzem S, Standl E, Jungmann E. In vitro activity of biosynthetic human diarginyl insulin. *Diabetologia* 1990; 33:65–71.

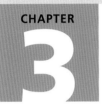

INSULIN GLARGINE: CLINICAL EVIDENCE

PHASE I AND PHASE II STUDIES	PRINCIPAL PHASE III/ III B STUDIES	META-REGRESSION AND META-ANALYSIS STUDIES

PHASE I AND PHASE II STUDIES

1021	p.93
Marbury	

2004	p.95
Matthews	

US	p.98
Raskin	

PRINCIPAL PHASE III/ III B STUDIES

3002	
	p.99
Massi Benedetti	
	p.102
Yki-Järvinen	
3012	p.104
Kacerovsky-Bielesz	
	p.168
Witthaus	

3006	
	p.106
Rosenstock	
	p.109
Fonseca	

4001	p.111
Fritsche	

4002	
	p.115
Riddle	
	p.121
Riddle	
	p.170
Johnson	

META-REGRESSION AND META-ANALYSIS STUDIES

	p.119
Yki-Järvinen	

	p.123
Rosenstock	

	p.123
Dailey	

KEY

1021	Study Number
p.93	Page Number
BOLD TEXT	Study published in peer review journals

PHASE IV STUDIES

4009

p.125
Standl

p.127
Standl

p.129
Fach

4013 p.131
Eliaschewitz

LEAD p.133
Pan

p.135
Rosenstock

SWITCH-pilot p.139
Schiel

LAPTOP p.141
Janka

OTHER RANDOMIZED STUDIES

p.143
Malone

p.145
Malone

p.147
Jacober

ALGORITHM COMPARISON STUDIES

AT. LANTUS

p.149
Davies

p.151
Lavalle-González

LANMET p.153
Yki-Järvinen

UNCONTROLLED OBSERVATIONAL STUDIES

Long Term

p.155
Schreiber

p.157
Schreiber

p.159
Fischer

Short Term

p.161
Klinge

p.163
Jungmann

p.165
Stryjek-Kaminska

p.166
Schreiber

TREATMENT COST

p.171
Al-Zakwani

p.172
Terrés

INCOMPLETE STUDIES

p.173
Seigmund

GOALAIC p.173
Pfeifer

p.174
Janka

p.174
Levin

p.175
Rosenstock

p.177
Raskin

OVERVIEW

The treatment of T2DM and prevention of its long-term complications has become an increasingly pressing challenge for clinicians worldwide. Traditional guidelines for the management of T2DM are designed to cope with the progressive nature of the disease and involve a step-up approach in which modification of diet and exercise in the early stages is promptly followed by treatment with blood glucose-lowering agents and then, as β cell function fails and glycemic control becomes more difficult to maintain, insulin therapy, in the form of basal insulin combined with oral agents and eventually a basal/bolus insulin regime, is introduced. This step-up conventional treatment paradigm that can take up to 10 years to introduce insulin therapy has been recently challenged by studies showing that the early addition of insulin therapy to oral hypoglycemic agents can safely and effectively improve glycemic control in persons with T2DM close to the currently recommended stringent glycemic targets.

Clinical studies show that the early introduction of basal insulin therapy in persons with T2DM results in a rapid improvement in glycemic control. Although it is desirable to reduce HbA_{1c} to as near normal as possible by titration of the insulin dose, this objective must be balanced against the potential for an increased occurrence of hypoglycemia. This has important implications for the choice of basal insulin. Until relatively recently, the only insulin preparations available for basal insulin supplementation were the intermediate-acting NPH (or isophane) insulin and lente insulin and the long-acting insulin, ultralente. NPH insulin is the most widely used, but with a peak of insulin activity 4 to 6 hours after administration, the risk of nocturnal hypoglycemia is considerably increased. Furthermore, its duration of action is too short to provide 24 hour activity with a single daily dose, which can make controlling blood glucose levels with this formulation difficult. In contrast, insulin glargine has a peakless and prolonged action for up to 24 hours, which approximates normal pancreatic basal insulin secretion. Insulin glargine has provided the first practical tool with the potential to facilitate and translate a new treatment paradigm of early insulin replacement to reach glycemic targets in T2DM.

In this section, we describe the clinical studies that describe basal insulin therapy in persons with T2DM, studies which compare NPH insulin and premixed preparations to insulin glargine. We review the randomized clinical trials, meta-regression and meta-analyses and observational clinical practice studies in persons with T2DM introduced to basal insulin therapy.

The critical role of the study design, and in particular the insulin titration algorithm used to achieve specific glycemic targets, are reviewed in the context of how these factors influence the study outcomes, especially with respect to the HbA_{1c} levels achieved. The ultimate barrier, hypoglycemia, is what determines the value of the HbA_{1c} achieved, otherwise all insulins can be adjusted to their maximum dose. Critical analyses of these factors are presented, highlighting the pharmacokinetic impact of the insulin in achieving the lowest HbA_{1c} with the least risk of hypoglycemia.

PHASE I AND PHASE II STUDIES

Evaluation of the safety, efficacy and tolerability of insulin glargine in subjects with impaired fasting glucose, impaired glucose tolerance or new-onset type 2 diabetes.

Marbury T, Schwartz S, Rosenberg M, Johnston P, Jariwala N, Shukla U, Becker R, Saoud J. *Diabetes* 2003; 52(Suppl 1):A451 Abstract 1955-PO.

Abstract

STUDY DESCRIPTION

This was a phase I, randomized, double-blind, placebo-controlled, parallel-group study to evaluate the feasibility of insulin glargine therapy in pre-diabetes and new-onset T2DM subjects, closely monitored as in-patients. Twenty-one subjects were randomized in a 3:1 ratio (insulin glargine:placebo) to receive either once-daily subcutaneous insulin glargine (n=16) or placebo (n=5) at bedtime. One subject in each treatment group withdrew and 19 subjects received study drug. Subjects were confined to study centers for 15 days, where they were subjected to a 2-day baseline and a 12-day treatment phase. A structured titration was employed to achieve the target FBG of 80 - 95 mg/dL (4.5 – 5.3 mmol/L). Exercise testing and assessments of counter-regulatory hormones were undertaken to assess potential disposition to hypoglycemic events.

OBJECTIVES

To assess the efficacy, safety and tolerability of insulin glargine in pre-diabetic subjects with normal glucose tolerance (n=3), impaired fasting glucose (IFG) or impaired glucose tolerance (IGT) (n=9) and in subjects with new-onset T2DM (n=9).

BASELINE CHARACTERISTICS		
	Placebo	Insulin glargine
Male (%)	20.0	62.5
Age (years)	54.6 ± 3.5	54.8 ± 9.7
BMI (kg/m²)	31.2 ± 4.0	30.7 ± 4.6
FPG (mg/dL)	114	110
Data are means ± SD		

STUDY DESIGN

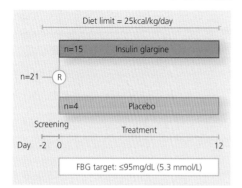

Figure 41. Design of phase I randomized study.

OUTCOME VARIABLES

Efficacy variables
- Daily FBG
- 24 hour 8-point BG profile
- BG before, during and for 3 hours after exercise
- Counter-regulatory hormones (epinephrine, norepinephrine and glucagon)

Safety variables
- Hypoglycemic events, defined as BG ≤ 50 mg/dL (2.8 mmol/L) or symptomatic events with BG ≤ 65 mg/dL (3.6 mmol/L)
- Changes in body weight
- All other adverse events

KEY FINDINGS

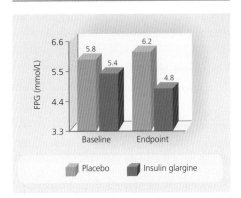

Figure 42. Baseline and study endpoint fasting plasma glucose levels.

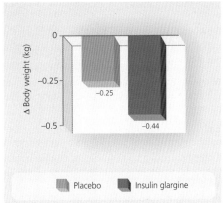

Figure 43. Change in body weight at study endpoint.

- Baseline to endpoint mean FBG levels fell from 96.6 ± 18.5 mg/dL (5.4 ± 1.0 mmol/L) to 85.6 ± 18.4 mg/dL (4.8 ± 1.0 mmol/L) with insulin glargine, but increased in the placebo group from 103.8 ± 9.3 mg/dL (5.8 ± 0.5 mmol/L) to 111.3 ± 17.5 mg/dL (6.2 ± 1.0 mmol/L)(Figure 42). The FBG target was achieved by 80% (12/15) of insulin glargine-treated patients.
- The 24 hour 8-point BG profile on days -1 and 12 showed reductions in mean BG concentrations throughout the day in the insulin glargine-treated subjects, compared to increases at most time-points in the placebo group.
- Mean BG levels following exercise were similar at the beginning and end of treatment (at days -1 and 13) in the insulin glargine-treated patients, but increased in placebo subjects.
- Changes in levels of counter-regulatory hormones between baseline and endpoint did not differ significantly between the two study groups.
- Five subjects reported 16 episodes of hypoglycemia. There were no episodes of nocturnal hypoglycemia. All episodes were mild and resolved rapidly on eating. There were no reports of exercise-related hypoglycemia in any subjects.
- Mean body weight decreased by 0.25 kg in the placebo group compared to 0.44 kg with insulin glargine treatment (Figure 43).
- No serious treatment-emergent adverse events were reported.

EDITORS COMMENTARY

This feasibility study in subjects with pre-diabetes who were glucose intolerant or who had minimal hyperglycemia shows that calorie restriction and treatment with insulin glargine can safely improve glycemic values to normoglycemia. Hypoglycemia was rare, mild and not related to exercise. This study provided the feasibility data that supported the rationale for the ongoing ORIGIN trial, described on page 17.

Additional References

1. Marbury T, Schwartz S, Roseberg M, Johnston P, Jariwala, N, Shukla U, Becker R, Saoud J, Deluca-Curran M. Evaluation of the safety, efficacy and tolerability of insulin glargine in subjects with impaired fasting glucose, impaired glucose tolerance or new-onset type 2 diabetes. *Diabetes and Metabolism* 2003; 29 (Spec No 2): Abstract 2209.

Safety and efficacy of insulin glargine (HOE 901) versus NPH insulin in combination with oral treatment in type 2 diabetic patients.

HOE901/2004 Study Investigators Group. *Diabetic Medicine* 2003; 20:545-551.

STUDY DESCRIPTION

This phase II, multicenter, open label study undertaken at 29 centers in Europe and South America enrolled persons with T2DM (n=256) who were poorly controlled on their current OHA therapy. Subjects had not received insulin treatment prior to study enrollment and were randomized (n=204) to receive once-daily injections at bedtime of either NPH insulin or insulin glargine, containing either 30 µg/ml [30] or 80 µg/ml [80] of zinc. The insulin dose was titrated individually to a target BG range of 72 – 126 mg/dL (4–7 mmol/L) over a three-week titration period, followed by a one-week maintenance period.

OBJECTIVES

To compare the efficacy and safety of two zinc formulations of insulin glargine to NPH insulin in insulin-naïve persons with T2DM who had failed to achieve good glycemic control on their existing OHA treatment.

STUDY DESIGN

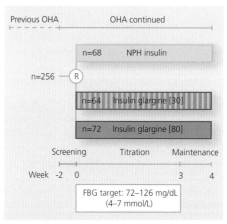

Figure 44. Design of phase II randomized study.

BASELINE CHARACTERISTICS			
	NPH insulin	**Insulin glargine [30]**	**Insulin glargine [80]**
Men (%)	57	58	64
Age (years)	59.2 (30–78)	58.9 (29–75)	60.0 (38–78)
BMI (kg/m²)	27.7 (20.1–39.0)	26.8 (19.8–34.2)	27.6 (19.6–35.3)
Duration of DM (years)	9.1	9.5	9.9
Duration of OHA (years)	7.1	7.5	7.7
FPG (mg/dL)	211 ± 56	223 ± 56	220 ± 49
HbA₁c (%)	9.5 ± 1.4	9.7 ± 1.5	9.7 ± 1.2
Data are means, with range or SD			

OUTCOME VARIABLES

Primary efficacy variable
• FPG

Secondary efficacy variables
• FBG
• BG profile – pre- and post-prandial (2 hours after breakfast, lunch and dinner), at bedtime and nocturnal BG at 03.00
• HbA_{1c}, fructosamine and free fatty acid levels
• Fasting serum insulin; fasting serum C-peptide
• Hypoglycemia: frequency of daytime events and nocturnal symptomatic and asymptomatic hypoglycemia
• Insulin dose
• Insulin antibodies; *E. coli* antibodies
• Local tolerance of injection

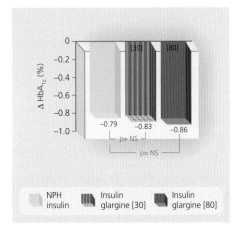

Figure 45. Change in mean HbA_{1c} measured at study endpoint.

KEY FINDINGS

• There were clinically relevant and significant (p<0.0001 in each case) decreases in adjusted mean FPG observed over the four-week study period in each of the three treatment groups (NPH insulin, -56 mg/dL (3.1 mmol/L); insulin glargine [30]: -61 mg/dL (3.4 mmol/L); insulin glargine [80]: 63 mg/dL (3.5 mmol/L).
• There were no differences between the three treatment groups in paired comparisons of mean-adjusted FPG (insulin glargine [30] compared to [80]; NPH insulin compared to pooled insulin glargine).
• All three treatments were associated with a significant decrease in HbA_{1c} between baseline and study endpoint, with no apparent difference between treatment groups (Figure 45).
• Levels of fructosamine, non-esterified fatty acids and fasting serum C-peptide were

significantly decreased in each treatment group but with no differences between treatments. Fasting serum insulin levels increased in a similar way.
• There was no significant difference in the incidence of at least one hypoglycemic event between the three treatment groups: NPH insulin (32.4%) vs. insulin glargine [30] (18.8%) vs. insulin glargine [80] (25.0%).
• A significantly higher number of patients receiving NPH insulin experienced symptomatic nocturnal hypoglycemia compared to the combined group of insulin glargine patients (19.1% vs. 7.3%; p=0.0123) (Figure 46).
• A significantly higher number of patients receiving NPH insulin experienced asymptomatic nocturnal hypoglycemia compared to the combined group of insulin glargine patients (5.9% vs. 0; p=0.0116)

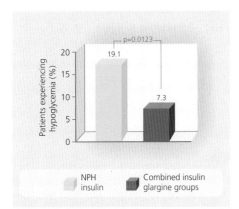

Figure 46. Frequency of symptomatic nocturnal hypoglycemic episodes.

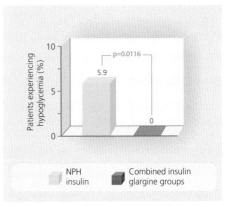

Figure 47. Frequency of asymptomatic nocturnal hypoglycemic episodes.

(Figure 47). No severe hypoglycemic episodes were reported.
- There were comparable increases in insulin dose (range 8 – 14 U) in each treatment group during the study.
- There were no obvious treatment effects observed in terms of antibodies to either insulin glargine or human insulin.
- Adverse events possibly related to study treatment were described in 2.9%, 4.2% and 4.7% of patients, respectively. An injection site reaction occurred in one patient in each treatment group.

Additional References

1. Matthews DR, Pfeiffer C. A new long-acting insulin (HOE901) demonstrates less nocturnal hypoglycaemia when compared with protamine insulin in a clinical trial. *Diabetologia* 1998; 41(Suppl 1):A245 Abstract 948.

2. Matthews DR, Pfeiffer C. Comparative clinical trial of a new long-acting insulin (HOE901) vs. protamine insulin demonstrates less nocturnal hypoglycaemia. *Diabetes* 1998; 47(Suppl 1):A101 Abstract 0394.

EDITORS COMMENTARY

This study, although small and of short duration, described the initial findings early in the research development program of the potential benefits of adding insulin glargine or NPH insulin to OHA, in persons with T2DM. Comparing insulin glargine to NPH insulin, insulin glargine was as effective as NPH insulin in reducing FPG levels and was well tolerated. But of the greatest clinical significance is the initial observation on the documented difference in the frequency of nocturnal hypoglycemia observed, both symptomatic and nocturnal asymptomatic events (defined as BG< 50mg/dL (2.8 mmol/L)), which were reduced significantly with insulin glargine compared to NPH insulin.

This study did not detect any evidence of a treatment effect on the development of insulin antibodies, or on antibodies to *E. coli*. The adverse event profile was as expected and similar between treatment groups. Only one patient from each treatment group experienced an injection site reaction.

No clinically relevant difference between the two formulations of insulin glargine was found. Therefore, the formulation containing 30 µg/ml of zinc was chosen for future investigation and ultimately as the final product formulation.

Abstract

The effect of HOE 901 on glycemic control in type 2 diabetes.

Raskin P, Park G, Zimmerman J, for the US Study Group of HOE901 in Type 2 DM. *Diabetes* 1998; 47(Suppl 1):A103 Abstract 0404.

STUDY DESCRIPTION

This was a phase II, multicenter, open label study of four weeks duration undertaken in North America. Patients with T2DM (n=157) who were poorly controlled on maximal OHA (sulfonylurea and/or metformin) therapy were randomized to receive once-daily injections at bedtime of either NPH insulin or insulin glargine, containing either 30µg/ml [30] or 80µg/ml [80] of zinc. The OHA therapy was discontinued. There was no significant difference in baseline characteristics.

STUDY DESIGN

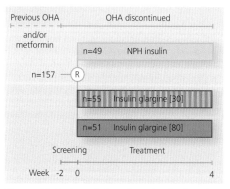

Figure 48. Design of phase II randomized study.

OBJECTIVES

To compare the efficacy, safety and tolerability of two formulations of insulin glargine to NPH insulin without concomitant OHA treatment in persons with T2DM who had failed to achieve good glycemic control on maximal OHA treatment.

OUTCOME VARIABLES

- Baseline to endpoint changes in:
  - FPG
  - HbA_{1c}
  - Fructosamine levels
  - Hypoglycemic episodes
  - Body Weight

KEY FINDINGS

- Comparing NPH insulin, insulin glargine [30] and insulin glargine [80], marked improvements in mean FPG over the four-week study period were described (-50 mg/dL (2.8 mmol/L), -47 mg/dL (2.6 mmol/L) and -41 mg/dL (2.3 mmol/L), respectively).

- There were no differences in the three treatment groups with respect to decreases in HbA_{1c}, fructosamine, and hypoglycemic events.

- Body weight remained unchanged in the treatment groups throughout the 4 week study.

EDITORS COMMENTARY

These results show no differences in outcome between the two formulations of insulin glargine; 30 µg/ml of zinc was chosen for future investigation and product formulation. Furthermore, this early phase II study also showed the potential benefits of insulin glargine or NPH insulin treatment in persons with T2DM who had failed on maximal OHA therapy. Comparing insulin glargine to NPH insulin, insulin glargine was as effective as NPH insulin in reducing FPG levels and was well tolerated.

This study did not appear to use a structured insulin titration regimen and despite stopping OHA therapy, all groups showed improvements in FPG levels, attesting to the important role of basal insulin therapy in T2DM.

PRINCIPAL PHASE III/IIIB STUDIES

Phase III registration studies

A one-year randomized, multicenter trial comparing insulin glargine with NPH insulin in combination with oral agents in patients with type 2 diabetes.

Massi-Benedetti M, Humburg E, Dressler A, Ziemen M, for the 3002 study group. *Hormone and Metabolic Research* 2003; 35:189–196.

STUDY DESCRIPTION

This phase III registration trial formed a key part of the regulatory submission for the approval of insulin glargine as therapy in persons with T2DM. The study, conducted in 57 centers in 14 European countries and South Africa over an initial period of 52 weeks, randomized a total of 578 patients and 529 patients completed the study. The study compared the efficacy and safety of insulin glargine and NPH insulin, both insulins given once-daily at bedtime. The study enrolled predominantly insulin naïve patients, but about 25% of patients had been previously treated with insulin. Previous treatment with OHA, which included any sulfonylurea and metformin, individually or in combination, continued unchanged. Insulin doses were titrated to a target FBG of ≤120 mg/dL (6.7 mmol/L).

The overall findings of the study were published in 2003 and included separate analyses of insulin naïve and insulin pre-treated patients and obese patients (n=529; Massi Benedetti et al., 2003). The efficacy and safety findings in insulin naïve patients alone were first described in 2000 (n=422; Yki-Järvinen et al., 2000). Once the randomized study was complete, the study was continued for a period of about forty months in a subgroup of patients (all had achieved HbA$_{1c}$ <10%) in which individually titrated insulin glargine at bedtime was given in conjunction with the existing OHA (n=239; Kacerovsky-Bielesz et al., 2002). The overall baseline characteristics of the whole population are shown below and are followed by separate descriptions of each of the publications.

OBJECTIVES

To compare the efficacy and safety of NPH insulin and insulin glargine in persons poorly controlled on OHA, with particular analysis of overweight subjects (BMI >28 kg/m^2).

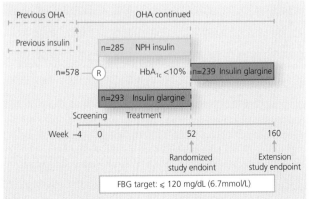

Figure 49. Design of phase III randomized study.

BASELINE CHARACTERISTICS		
	NPH insulin	Insulin glargine
Men (%)	54	53
Age (years)	59.4 ± 9.1	59.6 ± 9.3
BMI (kg/m²)	28.8 ± 4.3	29.3 ± 4.3
Duration of DM (years)	10.5 ± 6.0	10.2 ± 6.2
Duration of OHA (years)	8.3	8.3
FPG (mg/dL)	221 ± 58	225 ± 59
HbA$_{1c}$ (%)	8.9 ± 1.1	9.0 ± 1.2
Data are means ± SD		

OUTCOME VARIABLES

- Baseline to endpoint changes in:
  - HbA$_{1c}$
  - FPG
  - FBG
  - 24 hour BG profile.
- Frequency of confirmed (BG<50 mg/dL [2.8 mmol/L]) symptomatic and asymptomatic hypoglycemia

- Frequency of nocturnal (between evening injection and getting up) and severe (requiring assistance with BG<50 mg/dL or prompt recovery after oral carbohydrate, iv glucose, or glucagon) hypoglycemia

KEY FINDINGS

- Similar reductions in HbA$_{1c}$ between baseline and 52 weeks occurred in both treatment groups (NPH insulin: –0.32%; insulin glargine: –0.41%)(Figure 50).
- Similar reductions in FPG and FBG (range –2.6 ± 0.1 to –2.8 ± 0.2 mmol/L) occurred between baseline and endpoint in both treatment groups.
- During the treatment period, similar numbers of NPH insulin-treated patients compared to insulin glargine-treated patients experienced one or more episodes of symptomatic hypoglycemia (41% vs. 35%, respectively; p=NS)(Figure 51).
- However, more NPH insulin-treated patients experienced nocturnal hypoglycemia (24% vs. 12%, respectively; p=0.0002)(Figure 52).

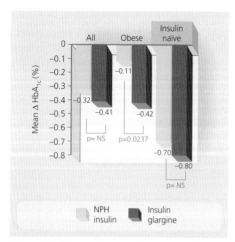

Figure 50. Change in mean HbA$_{1c}$ at study endpoint in all randomized subjects, obese and insulin naïve subjects. The insulin naïve findings (boxed) are derived from Yki-Järvinen et al., 2000.

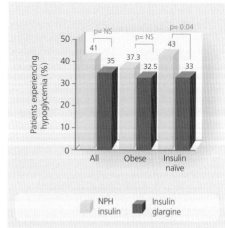

Figure 51. Frequency of symptomatic hypoglycemic events in all subjects, obese and insulin naïve subjects.

Obese subjects (BMI>28 kg/m²)
- On enrollment, 57% of patients were obese.
- There was a significantly smaller reduction in HbA_{1c} in the NPH insulin-treated group (-0.11 vs. -0.42%; p=0.0237) (Figure 50).

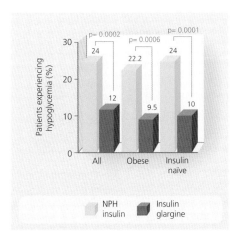

Figure 52. Frequency of nocturnal hypoglycemic events in all subjects, obese and insulin naïve subjects.

- Significantly more NPH insulin-treated patients experienced one or more episodes of nocturnal hypoglycemia (22.2% vs. 9.5%, p=0.0006) (Figure 52).

Insulin naïve vs. insulin pre-treated
- On enrollment, 25% of patients had been treated with insulin previously.
- Baseline values for glycemic control, FBG and FPG were higher and showed a greater decrease at study endpoint in the insulin naïve patients, as expected.
- In the insulin naïve patient group, one or more episodes of symptomatic hypo-glycemia occurred more commonly in the NPH insulin-treated patients, compared to insulin glargine (43% vs. 33%; p=0.04) (Figure 51) and nocturnal hypoglycemia was higher in NPH insulin-treated patients (24% vs. 10%; p=0.0001)(Figure 52).
- Insulin naïve subjects experienced a greater increase in body weight (NPH insulin: 2.34 kg, insulin glargine: 2.57 kg) compared to insulin pre-treated patients (0.63 kg and 0.16 kg, respectively).

EDITORS COMMENTARY

In this study conducted in persons with T2DM with unsatisfactory glycemic control, insulin glargine was as effective as NPH insulin when used in combination with OHA in reducing blood glucose both in insulin naïve and insulin-pre-treated subjects. Reviewing the complete study population, significantly fewer insulin glargine-treated patients experienced noctur-nal hypoglycemia (Figure 52). The authors indi-cate that, for those patients who reached the target FBG, fewer insulin glargine-treated patients reported episodes of symptomatic and nocturnal hypoglycemia compared to NPH insulin-treated patients. These results confirm and compliment the findings reported (Yki-Järvinen et al., 2000; page 102).

There was no difference in weight gain between the treatment groups, and the observed increase was small. As expected, insulin naïve patients experienced a greater increase in body weight compared to insulin pre-treated patients. This study suggests that insulin glargine may offer specific advantages for achieving glycemic control in overweight patients (BMI >28 kg/m²) compared to NPH insulin. The authors indicate that more insulin glargine-treated patients exhibited lower FBG and significantly lower HbA1c val-ues. However, the HbA_{1c} lowering effect was modest probably due to the relatively low insulin dose utilized in the study.

Less nocturnal hypoglycemia and better post-dinner glucose control with bedtime insulin glargine compared with bedtime NPH insulin during insulin combination therapy in type 2 diabetes.

Yki-Järvinen H, Dressler A, Ziemen M. The HOE 901/3002 Study Group *Diabetes Care* 2000; 23:1130–1136.

STUDY DESCRIPTION

This report was the first to describe findings from the registration study and reported the comparison of insulin glargine to NPH insulin exclusively in insulin naïve subjects.

OUTCOME VARIABLES

Primary variable
- Baseline to endpoint change in HbA$_{1c}$

Secondary variables
- Baseline to endpoint changes in:
  - FPG
  - FBG
  - 24-hour BG profile
- Frequency of confirmed (BG<50 mg/dL [2.8 mmol/L]) symptomatic and asymptomatic hypoglycemia
- Frequency of nocturnal (between evening injection and getting up) and severe (requiring assistance with BG<50 mg/dL or prompt recovery after oral carbohydrate, iv glucose, or glucagon) hypoglycemia
- Change in insulin dose
- Production of insulin antibodies
- Adverse events

KEY FINDINGS

- Similar, significant baseline to endpoint reductions in HbA$_{1c}$ were observed in each treatment arm (Figure 53). With NPH insulin treatment, the reduction was from 8.9 ± 0.1% to 8.2 ± 0.1% (p<0.001) and with insulin glargine, from 9.1 ± 0.1% to 8.3 ± 0.1% (p<0.001). In patients who reached the target BG of <120mg/dL (6.7 mmol/L), HbA$_{1c}$ level was further reduced in each treatment arm compared to baseline (p<0.001), with no difference between the two treatment groups (Figure 53).

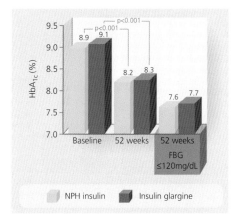

Figure 53 HbA$_{1c}$ levels at baseline and study endpoint. Findings in persons who achieved the fasting blood glucose target are highlighted.

- At the end of the 52 week study, BG concentrations were significantly lower in the insulin glargine treatment group both before (p<0.05) and after (p<0.01) dinner compared to the NPH insulin group (Figure 54a).
- Comparing NPH insulin to insulin glargine, the difference in before and after dinner BG concentration could be seen more clearly in those who reached the target FBG than those who did not (Figure 54b). Of note, of the patients achieving the FBG target, NPH insulin-treated patients experienced significantly lower nocturnal (03.00) BG levels (p=0.0005)(Figure 54b).
- The frequency of all and nocturnal symptomatic hypoglycemic events was significantly higher with NPH insulin compared to insulin glargine (p=0.04 and p=0.0001, respectively).
- In subjects who achieved the target FBG, the frequency of all symptomatic hypoglycemic events was also significantly higher in NPH-treated patients compared

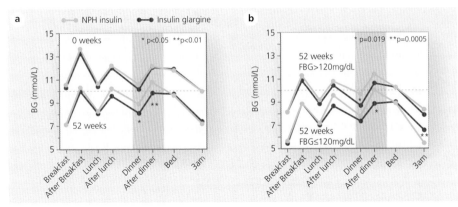

Figure 54. (a) 24 hour blood glucose profile at baseline (week 0) and study endpoint (week 52). Pre- and post-dinner blood glucose findings are highlighted. (b) 24 hour blood glucose profile according to fasting blood glucose target achievement. Pre- and post-dinner blood glucose findings are highlighted. (©2000 American Diabetes Association. *Diabetes Care* 2000; 23:1130-1136. Reprinted with permission).

to insulin glargine: all events 50.7% vs. 33.0% (p=0.027)(Figure 55).

- The frequency of symptomatic nocturnal hypoglycemia was significantly higher in NPH insulin-treated patients compared to insulin glargine if target FBG was achieved (28.8 vs. 12.6%; p=0.012) or not (21.4% vs. 9.0%; p=0.011)(Figure 55).
- At the study endpoint, the average dose of insulin glargine was 23 ± 1 U/day compared to 21 ± 1 U/day of NPH insulin.
- NPH insulin was more immunogenic than insulin glargine, with antibodies to insulin

significantly less prevalent in the insulin glargine-treated patients.

EDITORS COMMENTARY

This study provided important phase III randomized data after the introduction of a single bedtime injection of insulin glargine compared to NPH insulin. In this study, BG concentrations were significantly lower both before and after dinner with insulin glargine, reflecting differences in the duration of action of the insulin preparations. In those patients who achieved the FBG target of 120 mg/dL (6.7 mmol/L)), NPH insulin-treated patients experienced significantly lower BG in the early hours of the night, reflecting differences in the time-action profile of the two insulin preparations, and highlighting the effects of the typical peak of action of NPH insulin several hours after administration. This was reflected in the frequency of nocturnal hypoglycemic events, which was significantly higher in the NPH insulin-treated patients, for the same FBG concentration. Nocturnal hypoglycemia occurred more than twice as frequently in patients receiving NPH insulin. Of note, insulin doses were low, reflecting the relatively high FBG titration target, which explains the final HbA$_{1c}$ outcome.

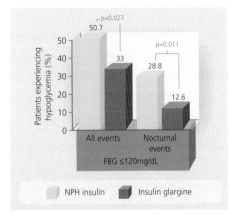

Figure 55. Frequency of hypoglycemic events in persons who achieved the fasting blood glucose target.

Abstract

Glycaemic control with insulin glargine in patients with type 2 diabetes is safely maintained in long-term exposure.

Kacerovsky-Bielesz G, Hirtz R. *Diabetes* 2002; 51(Suppl 1):A293 Abstract 1191P.

STUDY DESCRIPTION

This uncontrolled open label extension study was conducted in 45 centers in 11 counties and enrolled persons with T2DM all of whom had achieved HbA$_{1c}$ of <10% in the one year randomized registration study. Only patients who had been in the insulin glargine treatment arm were eligible to enter this uncontrolled study extension (n=239 in total).

OBJECTIVES

To assess the long-term effect (40 months) of once daily bedtime insulin glargine in conjunction with OHA in a subgroup of patients all of whom achieved HbA$_{1c}$ <10% in the randomized study conducted by the 3002 Study Group (n=239).

OUTCOME VARIABLES

- HbA$_{1c}$ levels, measured at the start of the randomized study (month 0), at the beginning of this extension study (month 12) and subsequently at months 24, 30, 33, 36 and 40.
- Incidence of symptomatic hypoglycemia (mild, moderate and severe).
- Adverse events, including injection site reactions.
- Antibody titers to insulin glargine, regular human insulin and *E. coli* proteins.

KEY FINDINGS

- The mean HbA$_{1c}$ level described in the randomized study (8.3% at 12 months) was maintained to study end in this patient group (8.4% at month 40) (Figure 56).
- Insulin glargine was associated with a low incidence of symptomatic hypoglycemia, which occurred in approximately 5% of cases. Around 3.3% of patients experienced

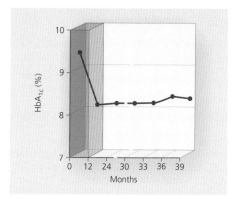

Figure 56. HbA$_{1c}$ levels during the 40 month study. Shaded area indicates the randomized study period.

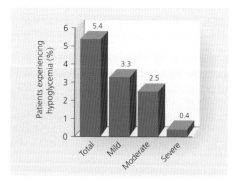

Figure 57. Frequency of symptomatic hypoglycemic episodes in insulin glargine-treated patients during the 40 month study.

mild, 2.5% moderate and 0.4% severe hypoglycemia (Figure 57).

- Baseline and endpoint measures of insulin antibodies were available for 208 subjects. In the randomized study, mean insulin antibody titers increased from 9.6% to 11.2% B/T. During this extension study, the level decreased to 10.4%. Increases of more than 20% occurred in 3.0% (n=8) of the insulin naïve patients.

- No additional weight gain was found with insulin glargine during this extension study, remaining approximately 2.0 kg above the baseline (Figure 58).
- Insulin glargine was well tolerated; there were no unexpected findings concerning the frequency and spectrum of adverse events. Whereas 5 systemic hypersensitivity events were recorded, none were considered to be treatment-related. No injection site reactions were reported.

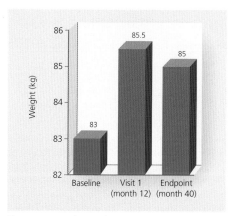

Figure 58. Body weight in insulin glargine-treated patients during the study.

EDITORS COMMENTARY

In this uncontrolled extension study, patients received extended insulin glargine therapy for up to an additional 28 months beyond the end of the original randomized study (combined maximum duration of insulin glargine therapy of about 40 months) mainly to test safety and the ability to sustain blood glucose-lowering effects. Insulin glargine doses continued to be individually titrated and treatment with OHA was continued throughout the entire study period. Patients attended for study visits every two months. Glycemic control was maintained without other adverse events, including injection site reactions and systemic hypersensitivity. Titers of insulin antibodies generally diminished over time.

Long term insulin glargine treatment maintained the improved levels of glycemic control and patients continued to experience low levels of symptomatic hypoglycemia. However, HbA_{1c} although improved from baseline, showed no further reduction, probably due to the conservative insulin dose and the lack of a more active insulin adjustment.

No definitive conclusions can be drawn from this uncontrolled study but nevertheless, the data on safety, antibody formation and durability of effect have clinical value.

Additional references

1. Massi-Beneditti M, Humburg E, Dressler A, Ziemen M. Lower incidence of nocturnal hypoglycaemia in patients with type 2 diabetes treated with insulin glargine compared with NPH insulin, given as a combination regimen with oral agents. *Diabetologia* 2002; 45(Suppl 2):A259 Abstract 804.

2. Yki-Järvinen H, Dressler A, Ziemen M. Comparison of insulin glargine (HOE901) vs. NPH insulin during 1 year of insulin combination therapy in type 2 diabetes. *Diabetes* 2000; 49(Suppl 1):A130 Abstract 529-P.

Basal insulin therapy in type 2 diabetes: 28-week comparison of insulin glargine (HOE901) and NPH insulin.

Rosenstock J, Schwartz SL, Clark CM, Park GD, Donley DW, Edwards MB. *Diabetes Care* 2001; 24:631–636.

STUDY DESCRIPTION

This phase III, randomized, open-label comparison of insulin glargine and NPH insulin was undertaken in 518 persons with T2DM at 59 centers in North America by the 3006 Study Group. A key feature of this study is that all subjects had received prior insulin treatment for more than three months without concomitant OHA prior to enrollment.

The prior insulin treatment was either once (n=100) or twice (n=409) daily, or more than twice daily (n=9) NPH insulin for basal supplementation. In addition, 328 patients had received concomitant regular insulin for postprandial glycemic control. Patients who had received prior NPH insulin as once-daily treatment (n=100) were the subject of an additional analysis (Fonseca et al., 2001, see page 109).

OBJECTIVES

To compare the efficacy and safety of insulin glargine and NPH insulin for basal insulin requirements in persons with T2DM on pre-existing basal (NPH insulin) alone or in combination with regular insulin regimens.

STUDY DESIGN

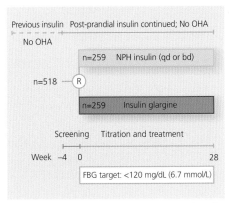

Figure 59. Design of phase III randomized study.

OUTCOME VARIABLES

Primary variables
• Baseline to endpoint change in HbA_{1c}

Secondary variables
• Baseline to endpoint changes in FBG.

BASELINE CHARACTERISTICS		
	NPH insulin	**Insulin glargine**
Men (%)	62.2	57.9
Age (years)	59.2 ± 9.9	59.5 ± 9.7
BMI (kg/m²)	30.4 ± 5.1	30.7 ± 5.0
Duration of DM (years)	14.1 ± 9.0	13.4 ± 8.3
Duration of insulin treatment (years)	8.3 ± 7.6	8.4 ± 6.9
FPG (mg/dL)	200 ± 77	191 ± 70
HbA_{1c} (%)	8.5 ± 1.2	8.6 ± 1.2
Data are means ± SD		

- Frequency of symptomatic (BG < 50 mg/dL (2.8 mmol/L)) and severe (BG < 36 mg/dL (2.0 mmol/L) and needing assistance by a third person to receive oral carbohydrate or intravenous glucose or glucagon) hypoglycemia
- Frequency of nocturnal hypoglycemia
- Baseline to endpoint changes in:
  - Body weight
  - Insulin dose
- Adverse events

KEY FINDINGS

- Comparing NPH insulin to insulin glargine, similar significant baseline to endpoint reductions in HbA_{1c} occurred in both treatment groups (mean reductions: 0.6 ± 0.1% (p=0.0001) vs. 0.4 ± 0.1% (p=0.0001) (Figure 60).
- FBG levels were similar at baseline in both NPH insulin and insulin glargine treatment groups and were reduced significantly in both treatment groups (Figure 61). Similar proportions of patients achieved the FBG target of 120 mg/dL (6.7 mmol/L)(27.1% vs. 29.6%, respectively).
- The occurrence of any symptomatic hypoglycemic event was similar in the two groups (66.8% vs. 61.4%). Severe hypoglycemia was more common with NPH insulin (10.4% vs. 6.6%; p=0.0553). Nocturnal hypoglycemia was 25% less frequent with insulin glargine after the initial titration phase of one month (35.5% vs. 26.5% p=0.0136)(Figure 62).
- Patients treated with insulin glargine experienced significantly less weight gain compared to NPH insulin treatment (1.4kg vs. 0.4kg; p<0.0007)(Figure 63).

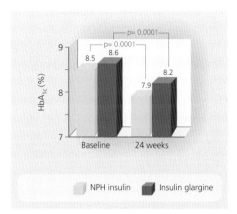

Figure 60. Comparison of mean HbA_{1c} levels at baseline and study endpoint.

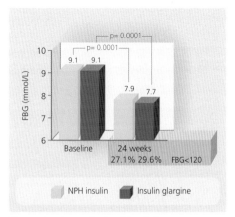

Figure 61. Mean fasting blood glucose concentration at baseline and study endpoint; the proportion of patients reaching target is shown in the shaded box.

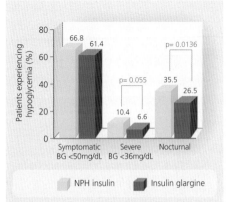

Figure 62. Frequency of hypoglycemia defined as symptomatic, severe and nocturnal during study.

EDITORS COMMENTARY

This study examined a group of patients who had previously been receiving insulin therapy with once or twice daily NPH insulin and in addition, approximately 60% of these patients had been receiving prandial insulin. The NPH insulin and insulin glargine treated patients achieved similar reductions in HbA_{1c} which remained sub-optimal at around 8% despite the conservative titration of insulin dose. This reflects the finding that only 30% of patients reached the target FBG, which may have been set too high at 120 mg/dL (6.7 mmol/L) to achieve a HbA_{1c} level of 7%.

With equivalent glycemic control, patients on insulin glargine had a significant reduction in the incidence of nocturnal hypoglycemic events. This finding may also account for the fact that the weight gain experienced by insulin glargine-treated patients was less compared to NPH insulin treatment.

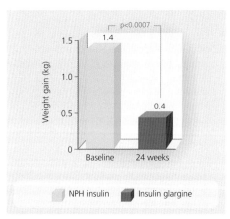

Figure 63. Mean body weight gain experienced by subjects during study.

Additional References

1. Rosenstock J, Schwartz SL, Clark CM, Edwards M, Donley DW. Efficacy and safety of HOE 901 (insulin glargine) in subjects with type 2 diabetes mellitus: a 28-week randomised, NPH insulin-controlled trial. *Diabetes* 1999; 48(Suppl 1):A100 Abstract 0432.

2. Rosenstock J, Schwartz SL, Clark CM, Park GD, Donley DW. Basal insulin glargine (HOE 901) in type 2 diabetes: A 28-week NPH controlled trial. *Diabetologia* 1999;42(Suppl 1):A18 Abstract 61.

Less symptomatic hypoglycemia with bedtime insulin glargine (Lantus®) compared to bedtime NPH insulin in patients with type 2 diabetes.

Fonseca V, Bell D, Mecca T. *Diabetes* 2001; 80(Suppl 2):A112 Abstract 449-P.

Abstract

STUDY DESCRIPTION

To examine the findings from the registration trial in more detail, the subgroup of 100 patients who had received once-daily NPH insulin for at least 3 months prior to entry into the randomized trial were subject to an additional analysis. Outcomes with respect to blood glucose levels and the occurrence of hypoglycemia were analyzed in those patients randomized to treatment with NPH insulin (n=48) and insulin glargine (n=52).

OBJECTIVES

To compare the effects of NPH insulin and insulin glargine on blood glucose levels and the frequency of hypoglycemia in a subgroup of patients from the registration trial previously treated with once-daily NPH insulin for ≥3 months.

OUTCOME VARIABLES

- Baseline to endpoint changes in:
  - FBG
  - HbA_{1c}
- Frequency of symptomatic (BG < 50 mg/dL (2.8 mmol/L)) and severe (BG < 36mg/dL (2.0 mmol/L) and needing assistance by a third person to receive oral carbohydrate or intravenous glucose or glucagon) hypoglycemia
- Frequency of nocturnal hypoglycemia

KEY FINDINGS

- Similar proportions of subjects achieved the FBG target of 120 mg/dL (6.7 mmol/L) comparing NPH insulin to insulin glargine (22.7% vs. 29.5%, respectively). The mean reduction in FBG was 20.3 mg/dL (1.1 mmol/L) and 17.1 mg/dL (1 mmol/L), respectively.
- A similar reductions in HbA_{1c} was achieved with NPH insulin (-0.44%) and insulin glargine (-0.35%) at study endpoint (Figure 64). The proportion of patients who achieved HbA_{1c} <7% (17.8% vs. 17.5%) and <8% (57.8% vs. 65.0%) was similar in each treatment group.
- Confirmed severe hypoglycemic events occurred more frequently with NPH insulin (31.3% vs. 17.3%; p=0.0017).
- The incidence of nocturnal hypoglycemia was 27.1% with NPH insulin and 15.4% with insulin glargine, but this was not significantly different (Figure 65).

BASELINE CHARACTERISTICS		
	NPH insulin	Insulin glargine
Men (%)	66.7	48.1
Age (years)	58.5 ± 9.8	57.3 ± 8.7
BMI (kg/m²)	29.24 ± 5.67	30.34 ± 4.41
Duration of DM (years)	12.7 ± 9.2	12.4 ± 10.0
Duration of insulin treatment (years)	6.9 ± 6.0	7.1 ± 5.8
FBG (mg/dL)	164 ± 38	169 ± 47
HbA_{1c} (%)	8.4 ± 1.0	8.4 ± 1.2
Data are means ± SD		

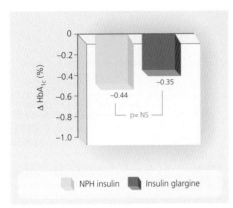

Figure 64. Comparison of change in mean HbA$_{1c}$ levels at study endpoint.

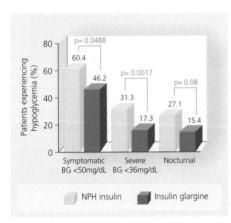

Figure 65. Frequency of hypoglycemia during study.

• The frequency of one or more episodes of symptomatic hypoglycemia was significantly greater in those treated with NPH insulin compared to insulin glargine (60.4% vs. 46.2%; p=0.0488) (Figure 65).

EDITORS COMMENTARY

In essence, this subgroup analysis of the phase III efficacy and safety study compared patients who were maintained on their previous treatment of bedtime NPH insulin to patients who were switched to insulin glargine. The key finding is that, in the presence of equivalent glycemic control, the occurrence of confirmed, symptomatic hypoglycemia was significantly lower in those patients switched to insulin glargine therapy. Of note, severe hypoglycemia was greater in the NPH insulin group, despite the limited number of patients in this analysis. This was a valuable sub-analysis of the main study indicating that significant reductions in confirmed symptomatic hypoglycemic events can be expected in patients switched from their evening NPH insulin to insulin glargine therapy. This article is now in press in *American Journal of Medical Sciences*.

Additional References

1. Fonseca V, Bell D, Mecca T. Less symptomatic hypoglycaemia with insulin glargine compared to NPH in patients with type 2 diabetes. *Diabetologia* 2001; 44(Suppl 1):A207 Abstract 796.

Phase IIIB studies

Glimepiride combined with morning insulin glargine, bedtime neutral protamine hagedorn insulin, or bedtime insulin glargine in patients with type 2 Diabetes: a randomised controlled trial.

Fritsche A, Schweitzer MA, Häring HU and the 4001 Study Group. *Annals of Internal Medicine* 2003; 138:952–959

STUDY DESCRIPTION

This open-label study, conducted at 111 sites in 13 European countries, randomized 700 persons with T2DM who had not achieved good metabolic control with OHAs. Of these, 695 patients were included in the full analysis set. The study consisted of a 4-week screening period before randomization, when patients were initiated on to, or were maintained on, treatment with glimepiride (3mg) ("one pill"). Patients were then randomized to concomitant insulin treatment for 24 weeks, either insulin glargine, injected in the morning or at bedtime, or NPH insulin at bedtime ("one shot"). The target FBG was ≤100 mg/dL (5.5 mmol/L) and the insulin dose was titrated using a pre-defined algorithm in an attempt to achieve this. The initial starting dose of insulin was calculated using the equation of Holman and Turner (FBG – 50 mg/dL ÷10 mg/dL), which was employed in the UKPDS.

STUDY DESIGN

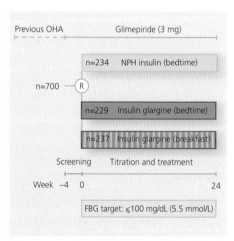

Figure 66. Design of phase IIIB randomized study.

BASELINE CHARACTERISTICS			
	NPH insulin (bedtime)	Insulin glargine (bedtime)	Insulin glargine (morning)
Men (%)	51.3	58.1	51.7
Age (years)	62 ± 9	60 ± 9	61 ± 9
BMI (kg/m²)	28.9 ± 3.9	28.7 ± 3.9	28.6 ± 4.5
Duration of DM (years)	9.3 (1-39)	8.2 (1-51)	9.0 (0-38)
Duration of OHA (years)	7.6 (0-38)	6.2 (1-30)	7.2 (0-38)
HbA$_{1c}$ (%)	9.1 ±1.1	9.1 ± 1.0	9.1 ± 1.0
Data are means with range or ± SD			

OBJECTIVES

To compare the efficacy and safety of a once-daily injection of insulin glargine (either in the morning or at bedtime) to NPH insulin, injected at bedtime, in persons receiving once-daily glimepiride and who were previously inadequately controlled by OHA alone.

OUTCOME VARIABLES

Primary variables:
- Baseline to endpoint change in HbA_{1c}
- Frequency of hypoglycemia (defined as symptomatic, severe and nocturnal)

Other variables
- Baseline to endpoint changes in FBG and BG profiles
- Insulin dose
- Body weight
- Adverse events

KEY FINDINGS

- Significant baseline to endpoint reductions in HbA_{1c} occurred in all three treatment groups. The reduction in HbA_{1c} was significantly greater for the morning insulin glargine group, compared to NPH insulin (p<0.001) and compared to the bedtime insulin glargine group (p=0.008) (Figure 67).
- Significantly more subjects achieved a HbA_{1c} level of less than 7.5% with insulin glargine given in the morning (43%), compared to NPH insulin (32%, p=0.017) and bedtime insulin glargine (33%, p=0.021) (Figure 68).
- The frequency of symptomatic hypoglycemia was significantly lower in the evening insulin glargine group (43%), compared to morning insulin glargine (56%; p=0.004) and bedtime NPH insulin (58%; p=0.001).
- There was a significantly higher frequency of nocturnal hypoglycemia with NPH insulin (38%) compared to insulin glargine, given either in the morning (17%; p<0.001) or at bedtime (23%; p<0.001) (Figure 68).
- Similar baseline to endpoint reductions in FBG occurred in all three treatment groups (Figure 69).
- Diurnal BG profiles showed a lower mean daily BG level with morning insulin glargine compared to evening insulin glargine (p=0.002) and NPH insulin (p<0.001) (Figure 70).

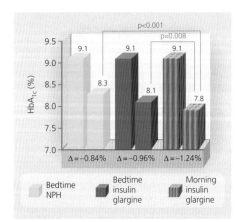

Figure 67. Mean HbA_{1c} at baseline and study endpoint. The change in HbA_{1c} is shown in the shaded box.

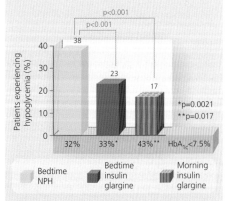

Figure 68. Proportion of patients experiencing an episode of nocturnal hypoglycemia; the proportion of patients reaching HbA_{1c} <7.5% is shown in the shaded box.

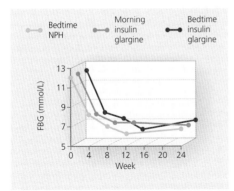

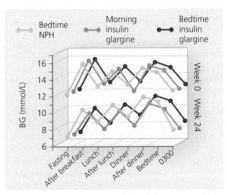

Figure 69. Fasting blood glucose profiles during the 24 week study period. (Modified from Annals of Internal Medicine 2003; 138:952-959. Modified with permission from the American College of Physicians).

Figure 70. 24 hour mean blood glucose profiles during the 24 week study period. (Modified from Annals of Internal Medicine 2003; 138:952-959. Modified with permission from the American College of Physicians).

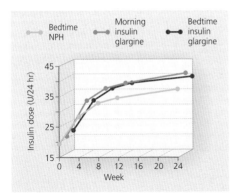

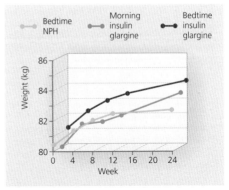

Figure 71. Profile of increasing insulin dose over the 24 week study period. (Modified from Annals of Internal Medicine 2003; 138:952-959. Modified with permission from the American College of Physicians).

Figure 72. Body weight profile over the 24 week study period. (Modified from Annals of Internal Medicine 2003; 138:952-959. Modified with permission from the American College of Physicians).

- Insulin doses at study initiation were similar and the baseline to endpoint changes did not differ significantly (Figure 71). During the study, the insulin doses increased from a mean (± SD) of 19 ± 11 U to 40 ± 24 U with morning insulin glargine, from 19 ± 11 U to 37 ± 22 U with bedtime NPH insulin, and from 20 ± 11 U to 39 ± 21 U with bedtime insulin glargine. The change of the insulin dose from baseline to endpoint did not significantly differ among the groups (p= 0.06).

- Body weight gain during the treatment period was modest and did not differ significantly between the treatment groups (p > 0.2) (Figure 72). Weight gain was 3.9 ± 4.5 kg with morning insulin glargine, 2.9 ± 4.3 kg with bedtime NPH insulin, and 3.7 ± 3.6 kg with bedtime insulin glargine.

- The adverse event profile was similar between the three treatment groups.

EDITORS COMMENTARY

This study tested a simple treatment regimen, sometimes referred to in the literature as the 'One Shot, One Pill' study (Rosenstock, 2004), in which the sulfonylurea, glimepiride, was combined with once-daily insulin, either NPH insulin given at night, or insulin glargine given either in the morning or at bedtime. All three insulin strategies achieved a significant reduction in HbA_{1c} compared to baseline. The morning administration of insulin glargine achieved the largest reduction in HbA_{1c}, a finding which may reflect the differences recorded in the diurnal blood glucose profiles with the different insulin regimens.

Although the total doses of insulin were basically similar, the higher proportion of patients achieving HbA_{1c} <7.5% with insulin glargine when given either in the morning or at bedtime reflects the lower frequency of hypoglycemic episodes associated with insulin glargine treatment compared to bedtime NPH insulin. This allows for more appropriate insulin adjustment and better 24 hour glucose profile. Nevertheless, the total doses of insulin were relatively low and the final FBG were above 100 mg/dL (5.6 mmol/L) with the final HbA_{1c} >7%. The lowest frequency of symptomatic hypoglycemia occurred with bedtime insulin glargine.

This "One Pill, One Shot" study is the simplest and easiest regimen for the initiation of insulin therapy in persons with T2DM. This regimen requires only a single self-monitored BG measurement each day. Insulin glargine treatment offers the patient the option of morning or bedtime administration according to their individual requirements. Further improvement can be expected with more active insulin titration to target FBG. We would also suggest that the addition of metformin to this regimen is worthy of consideration, potentially enhancing the insulin's blood glucose lowering effect and, as such, would be highly recommended in clinical practice.

Additional References

1. Fritsche A, Häring HU, Togel E, Schweitzer MA. Treat-to-target with add on basal insulin - can insulin glargine reduce the barrier to target attainment? *Diabetes* 2003; 52(Suppl 1):A119 Abstract 512-P.

2. Fritsche A, Häring HU, Togel E, Schweitzer MA. Insulin glargine as add-on basal insulin facilitates treat-to-target attainment. *Diabetes and Metabolism* 2003; 29(Spec No 2)Abstract 2215.

3. Schulze J, Peiker J, Schweitzer MA, Fritsche A, Häring HU. Predictors for a successful add-on therapy with basal insulin in patients with type 2 diabetes and secondary failure of oral antidiabetic drugs. *Diabetologia* 2003; 46(Suppl 2):A275 Abstract 794.

4. Busch K, Fritsche A, Häring HU, Schweitzer MA, Vesper I. Insulin glargine plus oral therapy in patients with type 2 diabetes allows flexible dosing and leads to improved metabolic control with less hypoglycaemia versus NPH insulin. *Diabetes* 2003; 52(Suppl1):A443 Abstract 1918-PO.

5. Busch K, Fritsche A, Häring HU, Schweitzer MA, Vesper I. Co-administration of insulin glargine with oral therapy in patients with type 2 diabetes allows flexible dosing and improved glycemic control with reduced hypoglycaemia compared with NPH insulin. *Diabetologia* 2003; 46(Suppl 2):A6 Abstract 10.

6. Fritsche A, Schweitzer MA, Häring H. Improved glycemic control and reduced nocturnal hypoglycaemia in patients with type 2 diabetes with morning administration of insulin glargine compared with NPH insulin. *Diabetes* 2002; 51(Suppl 1):A54 Abstract 220-OR.

7. Fritsche A, Schweitzer MA, Häring H. Improved glycemic control and reduced nocturnal hypoglycaemia in patients with type 2 diabetes with morning administration of insulin glargine compared with NPH insulin. *Diabetologia* 2002; 45(Suppl 2):A52 Abstract 149.

The treat-to-target trial: randomized addition of glargine or human NPH insulin to oral therapy of type 2 diabetic patients.

Riddle MC, Rosenstock J, Gerich J; Insulin Glargine 4002 Study Investigators. *Diabetes Care* 2003; 26:3080–3086.

STUDY DESCRIPTION

This open-label study, conducted at 80 sites in North America, randomized 756 overweight persons with T2DM and inadequate glycemic control (HbA$_{1c}$ 7.5 - 10%) to once-daily bedtime insulin therapy, either NPH insulin or insulin glargine. The study comprised a 4-week screening period followed by a 24 week titration and treatment phase. This was a proof-of-concept study, designed to test the "treat-to-target" hypothesis, namely that (1) the provision of a single bedtime dose of basal insulin therapy, in combination with continued OHA treatment and a forced, intensive and structured insulin titration algorithm to achieve FPG of ≤100 mg/dL (≤5.5 mmol/L), can attain the target HbA$_{1c}$ ≤7% and (2) the use of insulin glargine would be more suitable than NPH insulin in achieving this stated HbA$_{1c}$ target by reducing the risk of hypoglycemia. This combined objective is reflected in the primary outcome variable, of achieving the target HbA$_{1c}$ ≤7% without a single episode of nocturnal hypoglycemia. Thus, a key feature of this trial was the intensive, systematic titration of the NPH and insulin glargine dose (shown in Figure 73b) to reach HbA$_{1c}$ ≤7% while attempting to avoid nocturnal hypoglycemia.

STUDY DESIGN

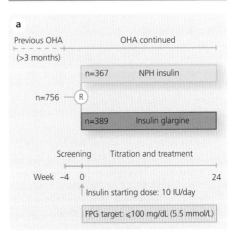

b

Start 10 U/day at bedtime

Mean FPG* (mg/dL)	Insulin dose** (U/day)
100–120	2
120–140	4
140–180	6
>180	8

* use means of preceding 2 days FBG values
** increase weekly only if no severe hypoglycemia and/or no PG values <72 mg/dL (4.0 mmol/L)

Figure 73. (a) Design of phase IIIB randomized study, showing trial design and **(b)** Forced weekly insulin titration algorithm.

BASELINE CHARACTERISTICS

	NPH insulin	Insulin glargine
Men (%)	56	55
Age (years)	56.8 ± 8.9	55 ± 9.5
BMI (kg/m²)	32.2 ± 4.8	32.5 ± 4.6
Duration of DM (years)	9 ± 5.6	8.4 ± 5.6
FPG (mg/dL)	194 ± 47	198 ± 49
HbA$_{1c}$ (%)	8.56 ± 0.9	8.61 ± 0.9
Data are mean ± SD		

OBJECTIVES

To compare the efficacy of bedtime NPH insulin and insulin glargine in achieving target glycemic control (HbA$_{1c}$ <7%) without the associated risk of nocturnal hypoglycemia in insulin naïve persons inadequately controlled by OHA.

OUTCOME VARIABLES

Primary variable
- The proportion of persons achieving target $HbA_{1c} \leq 7.0\%$ without a single instance of confirmed symptomatic nocturnal hypoglycemia (defined as PG of ≤ 72 mg/dL).

Other variables
- Baseline to endpoint changes in:
  - HbA_{1c}
  - FPG
  - Body weight
- The proportion of persons achieving target $HbA_{1c} < 7.0\%$ without the occurrence of nocturnal hypoglycemia
- The proportion of patients achieving FPG ≤ 100 mg/dL (5.5 mmol/L) without confirmed hypoglycemia.
- The frequency of symptomatic hypoglycemia including unconfirmed, confirmed and severe hypoglycemia.
- Within subject variability of FBG (between 7 sequential measurements).

KEY FINDINGS

- About a quarter more patients in the insulin glargine group reached the primary target of $HbA_{1c} \leq 7.0\%$ without documented nocturnal hypoglycemic events (33.2% vs. 26.7%; p<0.05) (Figure 74).
- Mean HbA_{1c} improved in both treatment groups to the target 7% (NPH insulin: 6.97%; insulin glargine: 6.96%).
- Mean HbA_{1c} fell steadily to a plateau level at 18 weeks in both treatment arms and was maintained to study end (Figure 75).
- The primary target HbA_{1c} of $\leq 7\%$ was reached by a majority of patients ($\approx 60\%$) in each treatment group (Figure 75).
- FPG declined to a plateau level at 12 weeks. Mean FPG at 24-week endpoint was not different in the insulin glargine group compared to NPH insulin (117 vs. 120 mg/dL (6.5 vs. 6.7 mmol/L), respectively) (Figure 76).

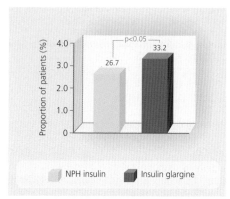

Figure 74. Treatment success expressed as percentage of patients reaching $HbA_{1c} \leq 7\%$ without symptomatic nocturnal hypoglycemia (confirmed by PG ≤ 72 mg/dL and/or meeting severe hypoglycemia criteria).

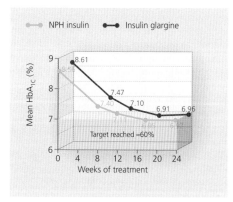

Figure 75. Mean HbA_{1c} levels during the study. Shaded area indicates the proportion of patients achieving target of <7%. ©2003 American Diabetes Association. Diabetes Care 2003; 26:3080-3086. Reprinted with permission.

- The mean weight gain (2.8 – 3.0 kg) was similar in both treatment groups.
- The FPG target (≤ 100 mg/dL) was achieved without hypoglycemia by fewer patients treated with NPH insulin compared to insulin glargine (15.9 vs. 22.1%; p<0.03).
- Overall, symptomatic hypoglycemic and nocturnal hypoglycemic events were

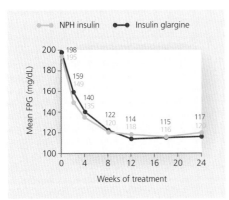

Figure 76. Mean fasting plasma glucose levels during the 24-week study. ©2003 American Diabetes Association. Diabetes Care 2003; 26:3080-3086. Reprinted with permission.

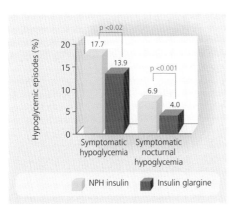

Figure 77. Episodes of symptomatic hypoglycemia during study.

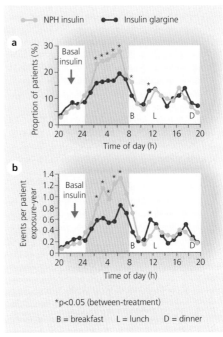

*p<0.05 (between-treatment)

B = breakfast   L = lunch   D = dinner

Figure 78. Distribution of hypoglycemia by time of day. The shaded area indicates the significant reductions in nocturnal hypoglycemia experienced by patients treated with insulin glargine compared to NPH insulin. (**a**) The proportion of patients experiencing at least one episode of hypoglycemia documented with plasma-referenced glucose ≤72 mg/dL (4.0 mmol/L). (**b**) The hourly hypoglycemia rates, expressed as events per patient-year at the same plasma-referenced glucose cutoff. ©2003 American Diabetes Association. Diabetes Care 2003; 26:3080-3086. Reprinted with permission.

significantly more common with NPH insulin compared to insulin glargine (Figure 77). Severe hypoglycemic events requiring assistance were uncommon in both groups (around 2.5% of subjects in each group).

- Reviewing the daily profiles of hypoglycemia shows that the occurrence of confirmed (PG≤72 mg/dL) nocturnal hypoglycemia was largely responsible for the significantly lower hypoglycemic rates compared to NPH insulin (Figure 78).

- There was significantly less within-subject variability of FPG between seven sequential fasting measurements during the study.

EDITORS COMMENTARY

This study proved that strict implementation of a structured but simple algorithm to titrate basal insulin dose to a FBG level of 100 mg/dL, when added to OHA, can restore HbA_{1c} levels to ≤7.0% in a majority of persons with T2DM. Both insulins reduced the HbA_{1c} levels in the majority of patients, but insulin glargine did so with a markedly reduced risk of symptomatic and nocturnal hypoglycemia. The fact that the level of patient adherence obtained was more than 90% suggests that this protocol can be easily followed.

This is a seminal study that can be translated to clinical practice, given the profile of the patient enrolled (overweight patients with HbA_{1c} of 7.5 – 10.0% despite OHA treatment), the simplicity of the treatment (only simple FBG measurements required, followed by once-daily dosing), and the low levels of the key side effect perceived as the main barrier to insulin replacement therapy (symptomatic and nocturnal hypoglycemia).

Additional References

1. Rosenstock J, Riddle M. Treatment to target in type 2 diabetes: consistent risk reduction of hypoglycaemia with basal insulin glargine as compared with NPH insulin in insulin-naïve patients on oral agents. *Diabetologia* 2002; 45(Suppl 2):A259 Abstract 805.

2. Riddle M, Rosenstock J. Treatment to target in type 2 diabetes: successful glycaemic control with less nocturnal hypoglycaemia with insulin glargine versus NPH insulin added to oral therapy. *Diabetologia* 2002; 45(Suppl 2):A52 Abstract 150.

3. Riddle MC, Rosenstock J. Treatment to Target study: insulin glargine vs. NPH insulin added to oral therapy of type 2 diabetes. Successful control with less nocturnal hypoglycaemia. *Diabetes* 2002; 51(Suppl 1):A113 Abstract 457-P.

4. Rosenstock J, Riddle M. Treatment to target study: timing and frequency of nocturnal hypoglycaemia. The value of adding bedtime basal insulin glargine over NPH insulin in insulin-naïve patients with type 2 diabetes on oral agents. *Diabetes* 2002; 51(Suppl 2):A482 Abstract 1982.

5. Rosenstock J, Riddle M, Dailey G, Gerich J, Mecca T, Wilson C, Bugos C. Treatment to target study: feasibility of achieving control with the addition of basal bedtime insulin glargine (Lantus®) or NPH insulin in insulin-naïve patients with type 2 diabetes. *Diabetes* 2001; 50(Suppl 2):A129 Abstract 520-P.

META-REGRESSION AND META-ANALYSIS STUDIES

The relationship between glycemic control and hypoglycaemia using insulin glargine versus NPH insulin: A meta-regression analysis in type 2 diabetes.

Yki-Järvinen H, Häring HU, Johnson E, Arbet-Engels C, Nguyen H, Zeger S, Riddle M.
Diabetes 2003; 52(Suppl 1):A149 Abstract 642-P.

STUDY DESCRIPTION

This meta-regression analysis was undertaken to determine the relationship between HbA_{1c}, FBG and hypoglycemia in a pooled group of 1785 patients with T2DM who had been treated with once-daily insulin glargine or NPH insulin within the context of three similar randomized controlled trials.

STUDY DESIGN

Subjects

The three randomized trials from which the data was pooled have common features, which includes the fact that all patients remained on OHA and were treated with once-daily insulin, either NPH insulin or insulin glargine, and that the treatment duration was similar (20 – 24 weeks), when outcome measures were assessed.

Data analysis

The data was analyzed (modeled) by fitting a Poisson regression with overdispersion in order to explore the relationship between the hypoglycemic events rates (events/100 patient years) from week 12 to study end (week 20 – 24) to determine the relationship between symptomatic and nocturnal hypoglycemia, with HbA_{1c} and duration of DM as covariates.

The overall mean hypoglycemic rates were compared using the ratio of mean rates from the model. The predicted mean HbA_{1c} levels were computed from a range of hypoglycemic rates based on the Poisson model. The frequency of hypoglycemic event rates between NPH insulin and insulin glargine was compared for a given FBG level.

KEY FINDINGS

Risk of hypoglycemia

- The regression modeling analysis demonstrated an increased rate of both confirmed symptomatic and nocturnal hypoglycemia with falling HbA_{1c} during treatment with NPH insulin and with insulin glargine (Figure 79).

- The model estimated that the mean number of confirmed hypoglycemic events was 23% lower in patients treated with a bedtime injection of insulin glargine compared to NPH insulin (ratio 0.77,

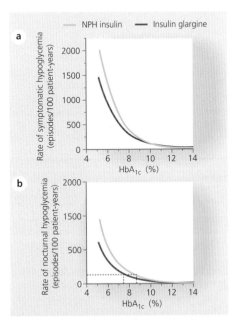

Figure 79. Meta regression findings showing relationship between (**a**) symptomatic hypoglycemia and HbA_{1c} (**b**) nocturnal hypoglycemia and HbA_{1c}. Figures used with permission of Prof H. Yki-Järvinen, MD, Helsinki, Finland.

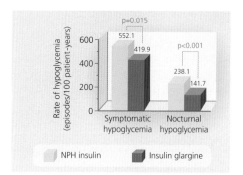

Figure 80. Rates of confirmed symptomatic and nocturnal hypoglycemia.

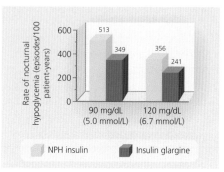

Figure 81. Rates of nocturnal hypoglycemia for a given fasting blood glucose

p=0.015; mean episodes: 420 vs. 552/100 patient-years respectively) (Figure 80).

- The frequency of confirmed nocturnal hypoglycemia was 39% lower in patients treated with insulin glargine compared to NPH insulin (insulin glargine:NPH insulin ratio of 0.61, p<0.001; a mean of 142 vs. 238 episodes/100 patient-years, respectively) (Figure 81).

EDITORS COMMENTARY

This regression analysis, using pooled data, indicates a lower frequency of symptomatic and confirmed nocturnal hypoglycemia with the use of bedtime insulin glargine compared to NPH insulin. At similar rates of both symptomatic and confirmed nocturnal hypoglycemia, a statistical and clinically significantly lower HbA_{1c} is predicted with insulin glargine compared to NPH insulin. Insulin glargine, therefore, will result in less hypoglycemic events than NPH insulin at similar levels of glycemic control.

In treating to a target FBG using intensive basal insulin treatment in T2DM, the use of insulin glargine over NPH insulin is consistently associated with a reduced risk of both symptomatic and nocturnal hypoglycemia. Therefore, correct evaluation of any study following the "treat-to-target" paradigm must carefully consider and assess the amount of hypoglycemia, not only as a major barrier but also as a major factor that can result in misleading HbA_{1c} findings. The findings of this analysis suggest that when the HbA_{1c} levels are similar in studies comparing NPH insulin and insulin glargine, it is conceivable that the increased rate of hypoglycemia with NPH insulin accounted for 0.5-0.9% of the HbA_{1c} reduction.

Predicted difference in HbA_{1c} for a given rate of hypoglycemia

- The model predicted that a HbA_{1c} level 0.44% lower could be achieved with insulin glargine compared to NPH insulin for the same rate of confirmed symptomatic hypoglycemia. This predicted reduction in HbA_{1c} is statistically significant across a wide range of symptomatic hypoglycemic rates (100 – 2000 episodes/100 patient-years) (Figure 79a).
- Similarly, at a chosen rate of confirmed nocturnal hypoglycemia, a HbA_{1c} level 0.87% lower is predicted with insulin glargine compared to NPH insulin (significant from 15 – 255 episodes/100 patient-years) (Figure 79b).
- At FBG levels of 90 or 120 mg/dL (5.0 or 6.7 mmol/L), the predicted levels of nocturnal hypoglycemia are lower in the insulin glargine-treated patients compared to the NPH insulin group (Figure 80).

Additional References

1. Yki-Järvinen H, Häring HU, Zeger S, Johnson E, Arbet-Engels C, Nguyen H, Johnson E, Riddle M. The relationship between HbA_{1c} fasting blood glucose (FBG) and hypoglycaemia using insulin glargine versus NPH insulin: a meta regression analysis in Type 2 diabetes. *Diabetes Metabolism* 2003; 29(Spec No 2):Abstract 2216.

Differences in HbA$_{1c}$ levels between insulin glargine and NPH insulin at equivalent incidences of hypoglycemia in patients with type 2 diabetes.

Riddle M, Arbet-Engels C, Nguyen H. *Endocrine Practice* 2004; 10(Suppl 1):48 Abstract 139.

Abstract

STUDY DESCRIPTION

This regression analysis was undertaken to specifically determine the relationship between HbA$_{1c}$ and hypoglycemia in patients with T2DM who had been treated with once-daily insulin glargine or NPH insulin within the "treat-to-target" randomized clinical trial (Riddle, Rosentstock and Gerich, 2003).

STUDY DESIGN

Subjects

This analysis included the 721 subjects within the "treat-to-target" trial (Riddle, Rosenstock and Gerich, 2003) who had completed 24 weeks of treatment of continuing their previous OHAs combined with insulin glargine (n=347) or NPH insulin (n=374).

Data analysis

The data was analyzed using Poisson regression to explore the relationship between the hypoglycemic events rates and the HbA$_{1c}$ level achieved with either insulin glargine or NPH insulin.

OBJECTIVES

A sub-analysis of data from the "treat-to-target trial" using a Poisson regression model undertaken to further examine the relationship between hypoglycemia and the HbA$_{1c}$ level achieved.

KEY FINDINGS

Primary findings

- At HbA$_{1c}$ levels between 5.6% and 7.8%, statistically significantly lower rates of nocturnal hypoglycemia and all hypoglycemic events occurred in subjects treated with insulin glargine compared with NPH insulin-treated subjects (p<0.05).

- At given rates of hypoglycemia, clinically significant differences in HbA$_{1c}$ levels associated with insulin glargine and NPH insulin therapy are predicted by the model. Under the conditions of the trial, at a rate of three events per patient-year, subjects are predicted to achieve HbA$_{1c}$ of 6.5% with insulin glargine and 7.5% with NPH insulin.

Secondary findings

- About three quarters of all patients with HbA$_{1c}$ ≤ 8.5% at baseline achieved target HbA$_{1c}$ ≤ 7.0% (NPH insulin, 75% vs. insulin glargine 74%).
- Of subjects who had a baseline HbA$_{1c}$ > 8.5%, 48% of insulin glargine-treated subjects and 45% of NPH insulin-treated subjects achieved HbA$_{1c}$ ≤ 7.0%.
- Of subjects who had baseline HbA$_{1c}$ ≤ 8.5%, 54% of insulin glargine-treated

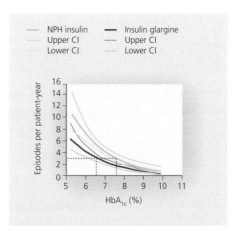

Figure 82. The model predicts similar rates of nocturnal hypoglycemia in patients treated with insulin glargine achieving HbA$_{1c}$ of 6.5% compared to those treated with NPH insulin achieving HbA$_{1c}$ of 7.5%. Figure used with permission of Dr M Riddle, MD, Oregon, USA.

subjects and 49% of NPH insulin-treated subjects experienced no episodes of nocturnal hypoglycemia (defined as BG ≤ 69mg/dL).

- Of subjects who had a HbA$_{1c}$ level at baseline > 8.5%, 38% of insulin glargine-treated subjects and 45% of NPH insulin-treated subjects experienced no episodes of nocturnal hypoglycemia (defined as BG ≤ 69mg/dL).

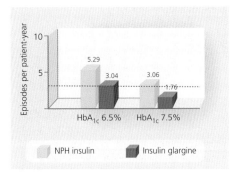

NPH insulin **Insulin glargine**

Figure 83. The model predicted similar rates (3.04 vs. 3.06 episodes) of nocturnal hypoglycaemia /patient–year, corresponding to HbA$_{1c}$ of 6.5% with insulin glargine and 7.5% with NPH insulin.

EDITORS COMMENTARY

Fear of hypoglycemia is a key barrier to reducing HbA$_{1c}$ levels in persons with T2DM. The "treat-to-target" trial showed that systematic titration of the dose of insulin glargine or NPH insulin resulted in 60% of insulin-naïve patients on OHAs achieving a target HbA$_{1c}$ ≤ 7%, with reduced levels of hypoglycemia in patients treated with insulin glargine.

The meta-regression analysis by Yki-Jarvinen and colleagues (2003) described on page 119 was undertaken in a larger number of subjects and utilized data from three studies, including the "treat-to-target" trial, and found that, at similar rates of both symptomatic and confirmed nocturnal hypoglycemia, a statistical and clinically significantly lower HbA$_{1c}$ was predicted with insulin glargine compared to NPH insulin. This present analysis of data from the "treat-to-target" trial confirms that for equal amounts of hypoglycemia, lower HbA$_{1c}$ levels are to be expected with insulin glargine.

References

1. Riddle MC, Rosenstock J, Gerich J. The treat-to-target trial: randomized addition of glargine or human NPH insulin to oral therapy of type 2 diabetic patients. *Diabetes Care* 2003; 26:3080–3086.

2. Yki-Järvinen H, Häring HU, Johnson E, Arbet-Engels C, Nguyen H, Zeger S, Riddle M. The relationship between glycemic control and hypoglycaemia using insulin glargine versus NPH insulin: A meta-regression analysis in type 2 diabetes. *Diabetes* 2003; 52(Suppl 1):A149 Abstract 642–P.

Confirmed lower risk of hypoglycemia with insulin glargine versus NPH insulin: a meta analysis of 2304 patients with type 2 diabetes.

Rosenstock J, Massi Benedetti M, Häring HA, Lin Z, Salzman A. *Diabetologia* 2003; 46(Suppl 2): A304 Abstract 879.

And

A meta-analysis of phase III/IIIb studies comparing insulin glargine with human NPH insulin in type 2 diabetes: severe hypoglycemia is less common with insulin glargine.

Dailey G, Riddle M, Massi Benedetti M, Fritsche A, Lin Z, Salzman A. *Diabetologia* 2003; 46(Suppl 2):A305 Abstract 880.

STUDY DESCRIPTION

These two reports describe a meta-analysis of the principal randomized multi-center studies of insulin glargine versus once- or twice daily NPH insulin in adults with T2DM. The "treat-to-target" study (Riddle, Rosenstock and Gerich, 2003) described on page 115 showed that patients achieved target glycemic control ($HbA_{1c} \leq 7$ %) with both once-daily insulin glargine and NPH insulin. However, the frequency of hypoglycemia, including confirmed nocturnal hypoglycemia, was higher with NPH insulin for the same level of glycemic control. This meta-analysis further examined the relative efficacy and safety of once-daily insulin glargine compared to NPH insulin, once- or twice-daily, in a large population of persons with T2DM.

STUDY DESIGN

In this standard meta-analysis, data from 2304 persons with T2DM from four comparative multi-center randomized clinical trials (Massi-Benedetti et al., 2003; Rosenstock et al., 2001; Riddle, Rosenstock and Gerich, 2003 and Fritsche et al., 2003) that compared NPH insulin, once- or twice-daily (n=1162), and insulin glargine once-daily (n=1142) was pooled. Patient demographics of the two treatment groups were essentially similar. The duration of the four studies was 24-28 weeks, with the exception of Massi-Benedetti et al., for which interim data recorded at week 20 was used.

KEY FINDINGS

HBA_{1c} and glycemic control
- Overall, the baseline to endpoint change in HbA_{1c} was similar for the two insulin regimes, that is insulin glargine (8.8 ± 1.1% reduced to 7.8 ± 1.3%) compared to NPH insulin (8.7 ± 1.1% reduced to 7.7 ± 1.2%).

Hypoglycemia
- The frequency of all symptomatic hypoglycemia was significantly lower with insulin glargine compared to NPH insulin, which was most marked with respect to nocturnal events (Table 7).
- The odds ratios for overall and nocturnal symptomatic hypoglycemic risk were significantly in favor of insulin glargine compared to NPH insulin (Figure 84).
- The time-of-day analysis of the pooled data showed that the reduction of hypoglycemia was largely observed during nighttime (Figure 85).

References

1. Massi Benedetti M, Humburg E, Dressler A, Ziemen M. A one-year, randomised, multicentre trial comparing insulin glargine with NPH insulin in combination with oral agents in patients with type 2 diabetes. *Horm Metab Res* 2003; 35:189–96.

2. Rosenstock J, Schwartz SL, Clark CMJ, Park GD, Donley DW, Edwards MB. Basal insulin therapy in type 2 diabetes. 28-week comparison of insulin glargine (HOE 901) and NPH insulin. *Diabetes Care* 2001; 24:631–6.

Hypoglycemia type	Insulin glargine	NPH insulin	p-value	Risk reduction
All symptomatic events	54.2%	61.2%	0.0006	11%
Confirmed (PG ≤72mg/dL [≤4mmol/L])	46.0%	53.3%	0.0004	14%
Confirmed (PG ≤56mg/dL [≤3.1mmol/L])	29.9%	37.0%	0.0002	19%
Nocturnal events	28.4%	38.2%	<0.0001	26%
Confirmed (PG ≤72mg/dL [≤4mmol/L])	23.9%	33.9%	<0.0001	29%
Confirmed (PG ≤56mg/dL [≤3.1mmol/L])	16.3%	23.1%	<0.0001	29%
Non-nocturnal events	49.6%	51.7%	0.4642	4%
Confirmed (PG ≤72mg/dL [≤4mmol/L])	40.1%	42.9%	0.2553	7%
Confirmed (PG ≤56mg/dL [≤3.1mmol/L])	22.8%	25.4%	0.1545	10%

Table 7. Meta-analysis rates of hypoglycemic events.

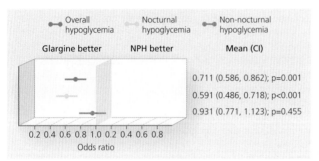

Figure 84. Odds ratio plot for symptomatic hypoglycemic events. Values are odds ratios with 95% confidence intervals.

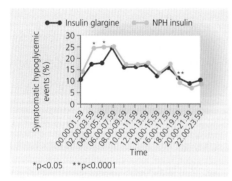

Figure 85. Meta-analysis time-of-day findings of symptomatic hypoglycemic events.

EDITORS COMMENTARY

These meta-analysis findings confirm that once-daily insulin glargine is associated with a reduced risk of confirmed symptomatic hypoglycemic events. The reduced risk of symptomatic hypoglycemia was particularly marked for nocturnal hypoglycemia with a risk reduction of up to 29% for events with PG≤72 mg/dL (4 mmol/L) and PG≤56 mg/dL (3.1 mmol/L). The lower hypoglycemic risk associated with insulin glargine compared to NPH insulin is clinically important when titrating basal insulin preparations to achieve target FBG concentrations below 100 mg/dL (5.5 mmol/L).

3. Riddle MC, Rosenstock J, Gerich J; Insulin Glargine 4002 Study Investigators. The treat-to-target trial: Randomized addition of glargine or human NPH insulin to oral therapy of type 2 diabetic patients. *Diabetes Care* 2003; 26:3080–6.

4. Fritsche A, Schweitzer MA, Häring HU. Glimepiride combined with morning insulin glargine, bedtime neutral protamine hagedorn insulin, or bedtime insulin glargine in patients with type 2 diabetes. A randomized, controlled trial. *Ann Intern Med* 2003; 138:952–9.

PHASE IV STUDIES

Incidence of nocturnal hypoglycemia in patients with type 2 diabetes is comparable when either morning or bedtime insulin glargine is co-administered with glimepiride.

Standl E, Maxeiner S, Schweitzer MA. *Diabetologia* 2003; 46(Suppl 2):A6 Abstract 11.

Abstract

STUDY DESCRIPTION

This European, open-label study conducted at 113 centers in 11 countries, initially screened 697 persons with T2DM who were poorly controlled by OHAs. Of these patients, 626 were randomized and 624 patients received treatment, with once-daily insulin glargine, administered either in the morning (06.00 – 09.00) or in the evening (21.00 – 23.00), combined with glimepiride, given orally before breakfast. Insulin doses were individually titrated using a structured algorithm aimed to achieve FBG levels ≤100mg/dL (5.5 mmol/L).

OBJECTIVES

To compare the frequency of nocturnal hypoglycemia following morning or evening administration of insulin glargine in combination with glimepiride (2 – 4 mg) in persons with T2DM.

OUTCOME VARIABLES

Primary variable
- Safety of therapy based on the incidence of nocturnal hypoglycemia (defined as symptoms occurring while asleep, after the evening injection and before rising in the morning)

Secondary variables
- All hypoglycemic events, symptomatic hypoglycemia (event with symptoms, possibly confirmed by BG <50mg/dL and not requiring assistance) and severe hypoglycemia (event with symptoms requiring assistance and confirmed by BG <50mg/dL or with prompt recovery after oral carbohydrate, intravenous glucose or glucagon).

- Baseline to endpoint changes in:
  - HbA_{1c}
  - FBG
  - Insulin dose
  - Body weight
  - Blood pressure
- All adverse events

STUDY DESIGN

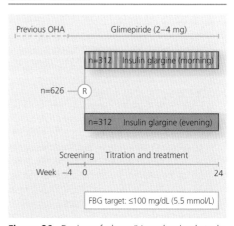

Figure 86. Design of phase IV randomized study.

BASELINE CHARACTERISTICS		
	Insulin glargine (morning)	Insulin glargine (bedtime)
Men (%)	54.5	54.5
Age (years)	62.1 ± 10.2	61.5 ± 9.6
BMI (kg/m²)	28.2 ± 4.0	28.7 ± 3.9
Duration of DM (years)	9.5 ± 6.1	10.3 ± 6.8
Duration of OHA (years)	7.08 ± 5.5	7.75 ± 6.0
HbA_{1c} (%)	8.82 ± 1.01	8.81 ± 0.98
Data are means ± SD		

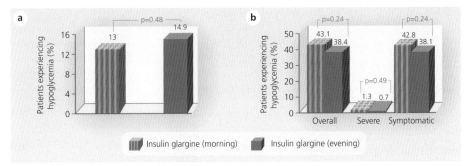

Figure 87. Frequency of hypoglycemia episodes during the study (**a**) Nocturnal hypoglycemia events. (**b**) All, severe and symptomatic hypoglycemic events.

KEY FINDINGS

- The proportion of patients experiencing nocturnal hypoglycemic episodes was similar for the morning and evening treated groups (13.0% vs. 14.9%, respectively) (Figure 87a). Of those patients who experienced nocturnal hypoglycemia, 51.3% (morning group) and 54.8% (evening group) had only a single episode.
- There was no significant difference in the overall incidence of hypoglycemia between the morning and evening treatment groups (42.8% vs. 38.1%, p=0.24, respectively) or severe hypoglycemia (1.3% vs. 0.7%, p=0.49, respectively) (Figure 87b).
- During the study, a similar significant reduction (p=0.042) in mean HbA$_{1c}$ from 8.8% to 7.2% occurred in both treatment groups.
- The mean reduction in FBG was similar in the morning vs. evening treatment groups (76.5 vs. 80.7 mg/dL, p=0.08).
- There was no difference in body weight and blood pressure between the two groups from baseline to endpoint.
- The mean, daily insulin glargine dose doubled over the study period from week one to study endpoint in both treatment groups (morning administration: 16.1 ± 8.1 increased to 34.7 ± 17.4 U; evening administration: 16.1 ± 7.9 increased to 32.4 ± 17.0 U; p=0.15).

EDITORS COMMENTARY

This large, open-label randomized multi-center study in patients poorly controlled on OHAs showed that the combination of insulin glargine and glimepiride improved overall glycemic control. There was no difference in HbA$_{1c}$ reduction between insulin glargine administration in the morning or at bedtime (–1.65% vs. –1.57%, respectively). Approximately 14% of patients experienced nocturnal hypoglycemia, half of whom had no more than one episode, and this was associated with a moderate body weight increase of 2 kg. The frequency of hypoglycemia, defined as any event, symptomatic events or severe events, was similar in the two insulin glargine-treated groups. The final mean insulin glargine dose reached at the end of the study period was similar in each treatment arm (morning insulin glargine dose: 34 U; evening insulin glargine dose: 32 U). It is conceivable that with the addition of metformin and higher insulin doses to attain FBG< 100 mg/dL, the target HbA$_{1c}$ could have been achieved. Nonetheless, a reduction to 7.2% is impressive, considering the relatively low insulin dose and the use of a sulfonylurea without a sensitizer.

Additional References

1. Standl E, Maxeiner S, Schweitzer MA. Morning versus bedtime insulin glargine in combination with glimepiride: no difference in incidence of nocturnal hypoglycaemia in patients with type 2 diabetes. *Diabetes* 2003; 52(Suppl 1):A134 Abstract 575-P.

Insulin glargine allows dosing flexibility in patients treated-to-target A$_{1c}$ of ≤7.0%.

Abstract

Standl E, Maxeiner S, Anderesi Z-K, Schweitzer M.A, HOE901/4009 Study Group. *Diabetes* 2004; 53(Suppl 2):Abstract 616P.

OBJECTIVES

This additional analysis of a European randomized, open label comparison of the efficacy and safety of insulin glargine administered in the morning or at bedtime in conjunction with glimepiride (2, 3 or 4mg) was undertaken to examine the group of patients (47% of total) who achieved target HbA$_{1c}$ of ≤7.0% to determine if target achievement influenced the rate of hypoglycemia.

OUTCOME VARIABLES

- Frequency of hypoglycemia:
  - Nocturnal hypoglycemia (defined as symptoms occurring while asleep, after the evening injection and before rising in the morning)
  - Symptomatic hypoglycemia (event with symptoms, possibly confirmed by BG <50mg/dL and not requiring assistance)
  - Severe hypoglycemia (event with symptoms requiring assistance and confirmed by BG <50mg/dL or with prompt recovery after oral carbohydrate, intravenous glucose or glucagon)
- Baseline to endpoint changes in:
  - HbA$_{1c}$

BASELINE CHARACTERISTICS		
	Insulin glargine (morning)	Insulin glargine (bedtime)
Age (years)	61.6 ± 10.6	60.7 ± 8.8
BMI (kg/m²)	28.2 ±3.9	28.8 ± 3.8
Duration of DM (years)	8.5 ± 5.2	9.4 ± 6.1
Duration of OHA (years)	6.3 ± 5.0	6.5 ± 5.2
FBG (mg/dL)	196	191
HbA$_{1c}$ (%)	8.6	8.5
Data are means ± SD		

- FBG
- Insulin dose
- Body weight

KEY FINDINGS

- Of the 624 randomized and treated patients, 292 (47%) reached target HbA$_{1c}$ ≤7.0%, with no difference in the proportion treated with insulin glargine in the morning (n=149/312, 47.8%) or at bedtime (n=143/312, 45.8%)
- Within this subgroup of patients who achieved target HbA$_{1c}$ of ≤7.0%, similar baseline to endpoint reductions in HbA$_{1c}$ were seen when comparing morning (8.6 to 6.3%, Δ=-2.3%) to bedtime administration (8.5 to 6.4%, Δ=-2.1%; p=NS)(Figure 88).
- Patients also achieved similar baseline to endpoint reductions in FBG. With morning administration, FBG fell from 196 to 114 mg/dL (10.9 to 6.3 mmol/L), Δ=-82 mg/dL (4.6 mmol/L) and with evening administration, from 191 to 108 mg/dL (10.9 to 6.0 mmol/L), Δ=-83 mg/dL (4.6 mmol/L); p=NS) (Figure 89).
- Baseline to endpoint increase in insulin dose was comparable between the two treatment groups (morning administration: 16.4 to 33.0 U compared to evening administration: 16.0 to 31.0 U; p=NS).
- Comparing morning to evening administration, the proportion of patients who suffered nocturnal hypoglycemic episodes (12.8 vs.16.8%, respectively p=NS), confirmed symptomatic hypoglycemia (49.7 vs. 42.0%, respectively, p=NS) and severe hypoglycemia (1.3 vs. 0%) was essentially similar (Figure 90).
- There was no difference in the frequency of nocturnal hypoglycemia episodes in patients with HbA$_{1c}$ >7% (13.8 vs.14.0%, n=324, p=NS) or in patients reaching target HbA$_{1c}$ ≤7% (12.8 vs.16.8%, n=292; p=NS) (Figure 90).

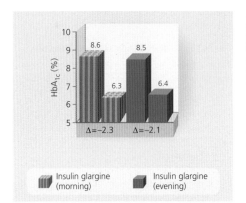

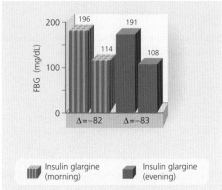

Figure 88. Change in mean HbA$_{1c}$ at baseline and study endpoint. The change in HbA$_{1c}$ (%) is shown in the shaded box.

Figure 89. Change in mean fasting blood glucose at baseline and study endpoint. The change in mg/dL is shown in the shaded box.

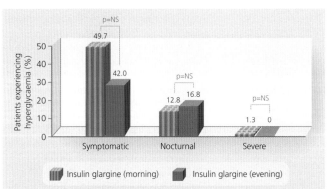

Figure 90. Proportion of patients experiencing episodes of hypoglycemia during the study.

EDITORS COMMENTARY

This study was undertaken in persons with T2DM (n=624) with poor glycemic control on OHAs (HbA$_{1c}$ 7.5–10.5%). Subjects were randomized to either insulin glargine in the morning (n=312) or at bedtime (n=312) to include glimepiride 2, 3 or 4 mg once daily and observed for a 24 week period. The insulin doses were adjusted using a forced titration algorithm to a target fasting blood glucose ≤ 100 mg/dl (5.5 mmol/L) and target HbA$_{1c}$ of ≤7%. This study was undertaken to analyze the results from patients who achieved the target HbA$_{1c}$ of ≤7% (i.e. 47% of target group).

This valuable sub-study of a European randomized study undertaken in patients with T2DM provides additional data to show that almost 50% of the patients treated with insulin glargine and glimepiride reached target HbA$_{1c}$ of ≤7.0% within 28 weeks, regardless of morning or bedtime administration of insulin glargine. This outcome compares closely with the findings of the "treat-to-target" study (Riddle, Rosenstock and Gerich, 2003), in which almost 60% of patients achieved the target HbA$_{1c}$ of ≤7.0%. Of note, patients achieving target glycemic control did not experience additional nocturnal hypoglycemic episodes compared to those that did not. There was no difference in nocturnal hypoglycemic events between the morning and evening insulin glargine treatment groups.

Efficacy of insulin glargine in type 2 diabetes: effect at different stages of disease.

Fach E-M, Busch K, Standl E, Schweitzer M.A, Anderesi Z-K, HOE901/4009 Study Group.
Diabetes 2004; 53(Suppl 2):Abstract 524P.

Abstract

STUDY DESCRIPTION

This additional analysis of a European randomized, open label comparison of the efficacy and safety of insulin glargine administered in the morning or at bedtime in conjunction with glimepiride (2, 3 or 4mg) was undertaken to examine if additional benefits are associated with the early introduction of insulin glargine. The stage of T2DM was reflected in the initial dose of glimepiride and therefore the efficacy and safety findings are described for three groups of patients receiving glimepiride 2, 3 or 4 mg once-daily.

OUTCOME VARIABLES

- Patient characteristics, including duration of T2DM and known duration of previous OHA treatment
- Frequency of hypoglycemia:
  - Nocturnal hypoglycemia (defined as symptoms occurring while asleep, after the evening injection and before rising in the morning)
  - Symptomatic hypoglycemia (event with symptoms, possibly confirmed by BG <50mg/dL and not requiring assistance)
  - Severe hypoglycemia (event with symptoms requiring assistance and confirmed by BG <50mg/dL or with prompt recovery after oral carbohydrate, intravenous glucose or glucagon)
- Baseline to endpoint changes in:
  - HbA_{1c}
  - FBG
  - Insulin dose
  - Body weight

KEY FINDINGS

- Comparing baseline characteristics, there was no difference between the three glimepiride dose groups in terms of age (63.3 ± 10.3 years), body weight (80.1 ± 14.0 kg), BMI (28.5 ± 4.1 kg/m^2) or C-peptide (1.5 ± 0.9 nmol/L; p=NS), but the duration of T2DM and the proportion of patients with a history of previous OHA treatment were significantly lower in patients on lower glimepiride doses.
- HbA_{1c} at baseline was significantly lower in the persons treated at lower glimepiride doses, but at study endpoint was similar in the three treatment subgroups (Table 8). Comparing the three glimepiride treatment groups (2, 3, or 4 mg), mean baseline HbA_{1c} levels were 8.5, 8.7 and 9.2% (p=0.0003) and mean endpoint levels were 7.1, 7.1 and 7.3% (p=0.6306)(Table 8).
- Similarly, FBG at baseline was significantly lower in persons at the lower glimepiride doses, but at study endpoint was similar between the groups (Table 8).
- Patients on lower glimepiride doses required a significantly lesser increment of insulin dose during the study and less insulin at endpoint (Table 8).
- Patients taking lower glimepiride doses experienced significantly less symptomatic (2mg: 30.7%; 3mg: 32.4%; 4mg: 50.0%; p=0.0414) and nocturnal hypoglycemia (2mg: 8.1%; 3mg: 5.7%; 4mg: 21.7%; p=0.0045).
- Patients taking lower glimepiride doses also experienced less weight gain at endpoint (2mg: 0.5kg; 3mg: 1.1kg; 4mg: 2.9kg; p=0.0001).

		Glimepiride dose			
		2 mg	3 mg	4 mg	p value*
HBA$_{1c}$ (%)	Baseline	8.5 ± 0.8	8.7 ± 0.9	9.2 ± 1.1	p=0.0003
	Endpoint	7.1 ± 1.0	7.1 ± 1.1	7.3 ± 1.3	p=0.6306
FBG (mg/dL)	Baseline	167 ± 35	179 ± 37	206 ± 49	p<0.0001
	Endpoint	115 ± 27	117 ± 29	123 ± 32	p=0.3064
Insulin dose (U)	Baseline	14.4 ± 6.8	14.8 ± 7.8	16.7 ± 6.8	p=0.2190
	Endpoint	23.5 ± 13.2	28.4 ± 15.5	34.1 ± 17.0	p=0.0012

* p values are between-treatment comparisons

Table 8. Summary of findings, showing baseline to endpoint comparisons of HbA$_{1c}$, fasting blood glucose and insulin dose.

EDITORS COMMENTARY

This study provides preliminary data on the value of early introduction of insulin in the management of T2DM. The findings are based on the premise that a low initial glimepiride dose reflects an earlier stage of the syndrome of T2DM, which seems clinically reasonable, but this is only an assumption. The findings suggest that, although glycemic control can be equally effectively restored in patients with longer disease duration who require higher doses of glimepiride, significantly higher doses of insulin are needed to achieve this, compared to patients initially on a lower glimepiride dose. The study also supports that the earlier introduction of insulin glargine may therefore result in significantly fewer hypoglycemic events and less weight gain, which is related to different insulin requirements.

This abstract presents a sub-analysis of the randomized trial, and the findings suggest future research opportunities to answer questions relating to the time of insulin introduction, in an attempt to obtain early good glycaemic control to prevent micro- and macro- vascular complications both in the short- and long-term ("metabolic imprinting").

Latin American clinical trial project on insulin glargine versus NPH insulin plus glimepiride in type 2 diabetes.

Eliaschewitz FG, Calvo C, Valbuena H, Ruiz M, Aschner P, Villena J, Ramirez LA, Jimenez J, Macêdo M, HOE 901/4013 LA Study Group. *Diabetologia* 2003; 46(Suppl 2):A272 Abstract 787.

Abstract

STUDY DESCRIPTION

This multi-center, open-label, randomized study was conducted in eight Latin American countries and enrolled 528 persons with T2DM and 481 were included in the intention to treat analysis. Patients poorly controlled on OHA were randomized to receive once-daily insulin glargine or NPH insulin at bedtime combined with a single, fixed dose of glimepiride in the morning, for a period of 24 weeks. Insulin doses were individually titrated according to the "treat-to-target" algorithm to achieve a target FBG ≤100mg/dL (5.5 mmol/L).

OBJECTIVES

To compare the efficacy and safety of once-daily, bedtime insulin glargine or NPH insulin combined with a fixed once-daily dose (4 mg) of glimepiride given in the morning in persons with T2DM.

STUDY DESIGN

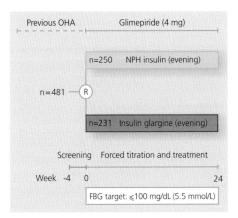

Figure 91. Design of phase IV randomized study.

OUTCOME VARIABLES

Primary measures
- Baseline to endpoint changes in HbA_{1c}

Secondary measures
- Frequency of confirmed nocturnal hypoglycemia, defined as BG<75 mg/dL (4.2 mmol/L) occurring during sleep
- Patients achieving HbA_{1c} ≤7.5%
- Baseline to endpoint changes in FBG

BASELINE CHARACTERISTICS		
	NPH insulin	**Insulin glargine**
Men (%)	38.0	42.9
Age (years)	57.1 ± 9.6	56.1 ± 9.9
BMI (kg/m²)	27.2 ± 4.0	27.3 ± 3.7
Duration of DM (years)	10.8 ± 6.4	10.3 ± 6.4
Duration of OHA (years)	8.9 ± 6.2	8.7 ± 5.9
FBG (mg/dL)	194.1 ± 56.6	201.8 ± 58.7
HbA_{1c} (%)	9.2 ± 0.9	9.1 ± 1.0
Data are means ± SD		

KEY FINDINGS

- Baseline to endpoint changes in HbA_{1c} were similar with NPH insulin (-1.44 ± 1.33%) and insulin glargine (-1.38 ± 1.32%), with no difference in the proportion who reached HbA_{1c} ≤7.5% (48% vs. 50.4%, respectively).
- At study end, a similar proportion of patients in the NPH insulin and insulin glargine treatment groups had achieved target FBG of ≤100 mg/dL (39.8% vs. 42.1%, respectively).

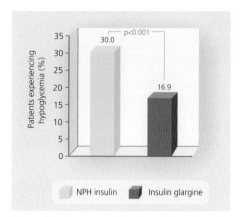

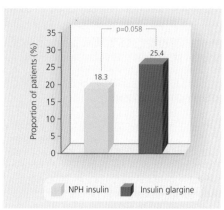

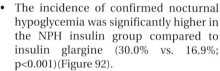

Figure 92. Frequency of nocturnal hypoglycemic episodes.

Figure 93. Treatment success in the intention to treat analysis data set (percentage of patients reaching HbA$_{1c}$ ≤7%, without symptomatic nocturnal hypoglycemia confirmed by BG ≤75 mg/dL (4.2 mmol/L)).

- The incidence of confirmed nocturnal hypoglycemia was significantly higher in the NPH insulin group compared to insulin glargine (30.0% vs. 16.9%; p<0.001)(Figure 92).
- The number of patients who achieved HbA$_{1c}$ ≤7.0% without occurrence of con-firmed symptomatic nocturnal hypoglycemia was not significantly different, comparing NPH insulin treatment to insulin glargine (18.3% vs. 25.4% p=0.058) (Figure 93).

EDITORS COMMENTARY

Comparative studies in European and North American populations have shown that insulin glargine is at least as effective at restoring glycemic control as NPH insulin, but information concerning the relative efficacy and safety of insulin glargine in the treatment of other ethnic and geographical groups, where cultural and dietary differences may have an impact, is not available. This Latin American study attempted to follow the insulin titration algorithm of the "treat-to-target" study with a similar study design (Riddle, Rosenstock and Gerich, 2003).

The findings show that a single, daily injection of insulin glargine combined with glimepiride, using the structured algorithm can reduce FBG and HbA$_{1c}$ with significant improvement in glycemic control in persons who were poorly controlled on OHA alone. Furthermore, compliance and consistency with the active insulin titration regimen remains a critical determinant of the final HbA$_{1c}$ achieved. This study suggests that the "treat-to-target" strategy is widely applicable with respect to geographic location.

Glycemic control and hypoglycemia in Asian type 2 diabetes patients treated with insulin glargine plus glimepiride versus NPH insulin plus glimepiride.

Pan CY, Bianchi-Biscay M, Chung K.-D, Won Kim K.-W. *Diabetes* 2004; 53(Suppl 2): Abstract 2043-PO.

STUDY DESCRIPTION

This randomized, open-label comparison of insulin glargine and NPH insulin was undertaken in 443 Asian persons with poorly controlled T2DM on their existing OHA therapy. The patients were randomized to either insulin glargine (n=220) or NPH insulin (n=223) at bedtime plus glimepiride for a period of 24 weeks. Patients' insulin doses were titrated according to a pre-defined dose titration regimen to a FBG target of ≤120 mg/dL (6.7 mmol/L). The titration commenced with an initial dose of insulin glargine of 0.15 U/kg/day, adjusted upwards by 2 units every three days until the target FBG of ≤120 mg/dl (6.7 mmol/L) was reached in the absence of hypoglycemia.

OBJECTIVES

To compare the efficacy and safety of a once-daily injection of insulin glargine to NPH insulin, both injected at bedtime, in persons receiving once-daily glimepiride and who were previously inadequately controlled by OHA alone (HbA$_{1c}$ from 7.5 - 10.5%).

OUTCOME VARIABLES

Primary variable
- Baseline to endpoint change in HbA$_{1c}$
- Frequency of hypoglycemia, including nocturnal and severe hypoglycemia

Secondary variables
- Baseline to endpoint changes in;
  - FBG
  - Mean daily BG
  - Nocturnal BG

STUDY DESIGN

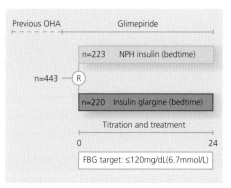

Figure 94. Design of phase IV randomized study.

BASELINE CHARACTERISTICS		
	NPH insulin	Insulin glargine
Age (years)	55.6 ± 8.7	55.6 ± 8.4
BMI (kg/m²)	25.1 ± 3.3	24.8 ± 3.1
HbA$_{1c}$ (%)	9.05 ± 0.84	9.02 ± 0.88
Data are means ± SD		

KEY FINDINGS

- Baseline to endpoint reductions in HbA_{1c} occurred in the NPH insulin and insulin glargine treated groups (-0.77 vs. -0.99%, respectively)(Figure 95). The difference between the adjusted means was 0.22% (p=0.0319), demonstrating non-inferiority between the two groups.
- Compared to NPH insulin, insulin glargine was associated with significantly fewer hypoglycemic episodes overall (1019 vs. 682; p=0.0036), including less severe hypoglycemic episodes (28 vs. 5; p=0.0257) and lower frequency of nocturnal hypoglycemic episodes (620 vs. 221; p<0.001)(Figure 96).
- Following the addition of insulin, changes in FBG and nocturnal BG were similar in both treatment groups. However, the reduction in mean daily BG was significantly greater in insulin glargine-treated persons compared to those receiving NPH insulin (-90.3 vs. -82.6 mg/dL (-5.0 vs. -4.6 mmol/L), respectively; p<0.05).

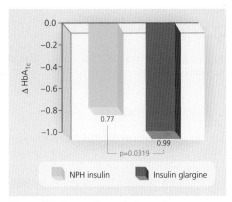

Figure 95. Comparison of change in mean HbA_{1c} levels at study endpoint.

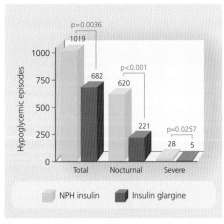

Figure 96. Frequency of hypoglycemia episodes during study.

EDITORS COMMENTARY

Most studies of insulin glargine have been restricted to European and North American populations, with the exception of one study based in Latin America (Eliaschewitz et al. see page 131). Information concerning the relative efficacy and safety of insulin glargine in the treatment of other ethnic and geographical groups, where cultural and dietary differences may have an impact, has been limited. This study in Asian persons with T2DM shows that insulin in combination with sulfonylurea results in clinically relevant reductions in HbA_{1c}. Insulin glargine was associated with a significantly lower level of hypoglycemia for a similar improvement in glycemic control compared to NPH insulin.

Triple therapy in type 2 diabetes (T2DM): Benefits of insulin glargine (GLAR) over rosiglitazone (RSG) when added to combination therapy of sulfonylurea plus Metformin (SU+MET) in insulin-naïve patients.

Rosenstock J, Sugimoto D, Strange P, Stewart J, Soltes-Rak E, Dailey G. *Diabetes* 2004; 53 (Suppl 2):Abstract 609P.

STUDY DESCRIPTION

This phase IV randomized, open-label comparison of insulin glargine with rosiglitazone was undertaken in multiple centers in North America. Insulin naïve persons with T2DM (n=217) with HbA_{1c} ranging from 7.5-11% and a BMI >25kg/m^2 who were being treated with a sulfonylurea plus metformin were randomized to add-on insulin glargine (10 U/day) or rosiglitazone (RSG) 4mg/day for a 24 week treatment period. This was preceded by a 4 week screening and titration phase prior to randomization when patients not currently on the maximum metformin dose were titrated to 2000 mg/day. The persons with T2DM then remained on this metformin dose unchanged during the treatment phase and the sulfonylurea dose remained unchanged throughout the titration and treatment phases. The insulin glargine dosing was adjusted according to a treat-to-target FPG of ≤100 mg/dL (5.5 mmol/L)(algorithm shown in Table 9). The rosiglitazone dose was increased from 4 to 8 mg/day at anytime after 6 weeks if the FPG remained above 100 mg/dL.

OBJECTIVES

To compare the efficacy and safety of insulin glargine and rosiglitazone as 'add-on' therapies in insulin-naïve persons with T2DM inadequately controlled on a combination of sulfonylurea plus metformin and changing to triple agent therapy.

STUDY DESIGN

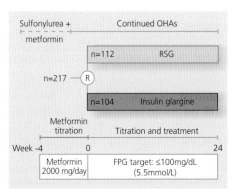

Figure 97. Design of phase IV randomized study.

OUTCOME VARIABLES

Primary variables
- Baseline to endpoint change in HbA_{1c}

Secondary variables
- Baseline to endpoint changes in:
  - FPG
  - Body weight
  - Total cholesterol (TC)
  - Low density lipoprotein (LDL)
  - High density lipoproteins (HDL)
  - Free fatty acids (FFA)
  - Triglycerides (TG)
- Proportion of patients reaching HbA_{1c} ≤8% and ≤7%
- Frequency of hypoglycemia, confirmed as BG <50mg/dL or severe hypoglycemia (event with symptoms requiring assistance and confirmed by BG ≤36 mg/dL or with prompt recovery after oral carbohydrate, intravenous glucose or intramuscular glucagon)

Mean FPG*, mg/dL (mmol/L)	Insulin dose increase** (Units)
≤100 (≤5.5)	0
≥100 and ≤120 (≥5.5 and ≤6.7)	0–2
≥120 and ≤140 (≥6.7 and ≤7.8)	2
≥140 and ≤160 (≥7.8 and ≤8.9)	4
≥160 and ≤180 (≥8.9 and ≤10)	6
≥180 (≥10)	8

*Titrated weekly according to self monitored plasma glucose values (SMBG) using a plasma referenced blood glucose meter for the last 2 consecutive days and no severe hypoglycemia or SMBG of <72 mg/dL (<4 mmol/L).
** Insulin glargine was initiated at a starting dose of 10 U per day.
Note: patients often did not get insulin increments if fasting plasma glucose was 100-120 mg/dL.

Table 9. The forced insulin titration schedule employed.

- Treatment costs, based on resource use with unit-cost estimates from secondary data sources, including study medications (average wholesale costs expressed in 2002 $US), syringe use, glucose testing supplies and liver function tests. Analyses were conducted on observed data only and not adjusted for between-treatment groups differences in the duration of treatment)
- All adverse events

KEY FINDINGS

- The decrease in HbA_{1c} from baseline to endpoint was similar for both RSG and insulin glargine (−1.51 vs. -1.66%; p=0.1446) (Figure 98). However, the reduction in HbA_{1c} was significantly greater for insulin glargine-treated patients with baseline HbA_{1c} of ≥9.5%.
- Similar proportions of insulin glargine and rosiglitazone-treated patients reached HbA_{1c} of ≤8% (92.3% vs. 83.0%, respectively) and target HbA_{1c} of 7% (48.1% vs. 49.1%, respectively, p=NS)(Figure 98).
- More of the patients who had required an initial metformin titration during the 4-week screening period reached target HbA_{1c} with insulin glargine compared to rosiglitazone (66 vs. 42%, p=0.0226).

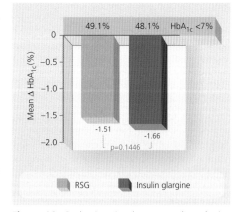

Figure 98. Reductions in HbA_{1c} at study endpoint. The proportion of patients achieving target HbA_{1c} of <7% are shown in the shaded box.

- At study end, the decrease in FPG was significant in both treatment groups, but a greater reduction was described in patients treated with insulin glargine compared to rosiglitazone (reductions: −64.9 vs. −46.3 mg/dL [−3.60 vs. −2.57 mmol/L], respectively; p=0.001)(Figure 99).
- Rosiglitazone-treated patients experienced a significantly greater increase in

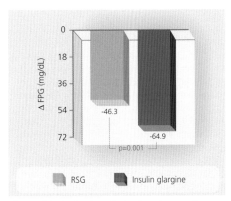

Figure 99. Reductions in fasting plasma glucose at study endpoint.

weight compared to insulin glargine treatment (3.0 ± 0.4 kg vs. 1.7 ± 0.4 kg, respectively; p=0.02) over the 24 week treatment period.

• Patients in the insulin glargine group demonstrated a significant improvement from baseline to endpoint (p <0.01) in TC (Δ=–4.2%), FFA (Δ=–22.4%) and TG (Δ=–15.0%), whereas patients in the rosiglitazone treatment group demonstrated significant increases (p <0.0005) in TC (+11.2%), LDL (+17.0%) and LDL/HDL ratio (+14.7%). The RSG group had significant improvements in HDL from baseline to endpoint (+4.8%) and FFA levels for insulin glargine (Δ14.6%, both p<0.025).

• Overall, the frequency of hypoglycemia was similar between the treatment groups, however confirmed symptomatic nocturnal hypoglycemic events (<50mg/dL, 2.8 mmol/L) were more evident with insulin glargine (24.8 vs. 12.5%, p<0.02), but there were numerically more severe hypoglycemic events with rosiglitazone (n=8 vs. 3, respectively).

• Rosiglitazone-treated patients experienced more adverse reactions (28.6 vs. 6.7%; p=0.0001) including the presence of peripheral edema in 12.5 % and none with insulin glargine.

• Mean insulin glargine dose increased from the initial dose of 10 units /day at baseline to 38.5 ± 26.5 U/day at endpoint.

• Insulin glargine treatment saved $397/patient compared to rosiglitazone over the 24 week study.

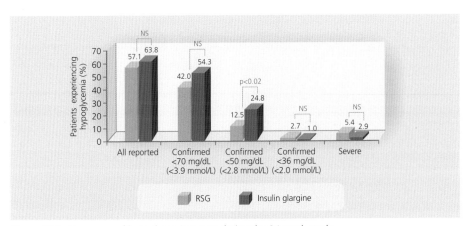

Figure 100. Frequency of hypoglycemic events during the 24 week study.

EDITORS COMMENTARY

The combination therapy of a sulfonylurea plus metformin remains a common standard regimen for managing T2DM. Additional therapy will be required by an increasing number of subjects with increasing duration of T2DM to achieve target glycemic control. In this study, the addition of insulin glargine resulted in better FPG with a similar hypoglycemic profile compared to rosiglitazone, and was associated with a superior adverse events profile. In addition, insulin glargine patients experienced significantly less weight gain with an improved lipid profile, and no episodes of peripheral edema. These benefits of insulin glargine were achieved at substantially reduced cost compared to rosiglitazone. Given that the algorithm used to increase the insulin glargine dose was less aggressive than that employed in the "treat-to-target" study, it is conceivable that even greater glycemic benefits could be achieved with a more intensive titration algorithm.

Quality of glycemic control and well-being of patients with type 2 diabetes mellitus after switching from conventional insulin therapy to once-daily insulin glargine in combination with oral anti-diabetic drugs – SWITCH Pilot, a prospective randomized trial.

Schiel R, Schweitzer MA, Müller UA. *Diabetologia* 2003; 46(Suppl 2):A272 Abstract 788.

Abstract

STUDY DESCRIPTION

This is a randomized parallel group, single center pilot study involving 52 persons with poorly controlled T2DM (HbA$_{1c}$>7.8%) on twice-daily pre-mixed NPH insulin (30/70 or 25/75 – conventional insulin therapy, CIT). Patients were randomized to receive one of three treatments: insulin glargine (morning) and glimepiride [Group A], insulin glargine (morning) and glimepiride plus metformin [Group B], or continued CIT with no OHA [Group C] for 16 weeks, preceded by a 4 week run-in phase, during which the previous insulin therapy was continued prior to randomization.

STUDY DESIGN

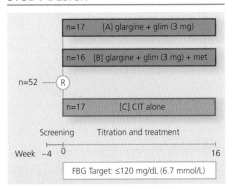

Figure 101. Design of phase IV randomized study.

OBJECTIVES

To determine the efficacy and safety of a morning dose of insulin glargine in conjunction with OHA (glimepiride alone or with metformin) compared to CIT, consisting of twice-daily pre-mixed insulin monotherapy, in persons with T2DM poorly controlled on their current therapy.

OUTCOME VARIABLES

- Baseline to endpoint change in:
  - HbA$_{1c}$
  - FBG
- 24 hour BG profile (FBG pre-lunch, pre-dinner, bedtime and at 03.00)
- Episodes of confirmed hypoglycemia documented by the patient (BG<60 mg/dL (3.3 mmol/L)) classified as symptomatic, asymptomatic, requiring assistance (BG<36 mg/dL (2.0 mmol/L) or improvement after oral carbohydrate) and severe (unconscious and requiring injection of glucose or glucagon)
- Baseline to endpoint change in:
  - Body weight
  - BMI
  - Blood pressure
  - Laboratory parameters
  - Treatment satisfaction.
- Adverse events

BASELINE CHARACTERISTICS			
	Group A	Group B	Group C
Age (years)	61.7 ± 10.7	65.4 ± 8.5	69.8 ± 6.4
BMI (kg/m²)	32.2 ± 3.0	31.2 ± 2.8	30.9 ± 2.9
Duration of DM (years)	15.3 ±8.4	14.2 ± 8.0	16.3 ± 6.7
Duration of insulin therapy (years)	3.8 ± 1.9	4.3 ± 1.7	4.3 ± 1.4
FBG (mg/dL)	158	171	153
HbA$_{1c}$ (%)	8.2 ± 0.7	8.1 ± 0.9	8.1 ± 0.8
Data are means ± SD			

KEY FINDINGS

- A significant reduction in HbA_{1c} levels occurred between baseline and endpoint in treatment groups A (- 0.4%; p=0.0128) and B (- 0.7%; p=0.0057), but not C (- 0.3%; p=0.3), (Figure 102a).
- Significant baseline to endpoint reductions in FBG occurred in the three treatment groups (Figure 102b). There was no difference in the proportion of patients who achieved a FBG<100 mg/dL.
- There was no significant difference in the frequency of symptomatic hypoglycemia

EDITORS COMMENTARY

This pilot study provides preliminary evidence or "proof of concept" that patients with long duration of T2DM on conventional insulin monotherapy can still respond to a simpler basal insulin regimen in combination with OHA, especially when used in combination with a structured basal insulin titration. Patients on twice-daily pre-mixed insulin are not necessarily "stuck" on this regimen. The potential exists for these patients to switch to easier, more flexible regimens with insulin glargine and oral agents. Compared with CIT using premixed insulin given twice-daily, insulin glargine given in conjunction with OHA provides equally effective glycemic control, but with a reduction in the required daily insulin dose. However, the target FBG was ≤120 mg/dL and it is conceivable that a target ≤100 mg/dL would have resulted in better HbA_{1c} reduction and higher insulin dose. Insulin glargine therapy had high acceptance with patients, with up to 88% choosing to remain on insulin glargine therapy at trial-end.

Although not large, this study provides insight into the glycemic outcomes after switching to insulin glargine. Future studies will need to investigate the optimal therapy for these patients, in particular, the use of structured titration regimens like "treat-to-target". The introduction of prandial short-acting insulin analogs in a progressive systematic fashion according to BG profiles will result in more flexible physiological regimens for these patients.

between the treatment groups. There were no hypoglycemic events regarded as severe or requiring assistance.

- At the study endpoint, there were no significant differences in patient well-being and treatment satisfaction scores (A: 31.6 ± 7.6; B: 32.6 ± 5.0; C: 30.9 ± 6.1). Most patients continued their randomized therapy.

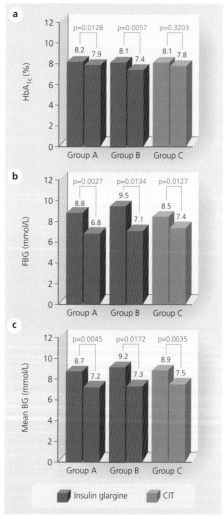

Figure 102. (**a**) Baseline to endpoint changes in HbA_{1c}. (**b**) Baseline to endpoint changes in fasting blood glucose.(**c**) Baseline to endpoint changes in mean blood glucose.

Starting insulin for type 2 diabetes with insulin glargine added to oral agents vs. twice-daily premixed insulin alone.

Janka H, Plewe G, Kliebe-Frisch C, Schweitzer M.A, Yki-Järvinen H. *Diabetes* 2004; 53(Suppl 2):Abstract 548-P.

STUDY DESCRIPTION

This phase IV randomized, open-label trial (known as "LAPTOP"), was conducted in multiple international centers in Europe (66). Insulin naïve subjects with T2DM (n=364), inadequately controlled on their existing OHA treatment (glimepiride or other sulfonylurea plus metformin therapy), with mean FBG >120mg/dL (6.7 mmol/L) and HbA_{1c} at entry ranging from 7.5-10.5% were randomized to insulin glargine given once daily in the morning with continued OHA therapy or alternatively to premixed insulin (30% regular soluble human insulin, 70% NPH insulin (PreMix) twice-daily, discontinuing all OHA therapy, for a treatment period of 24 weeks. The insulin glargine dose was titrated to a target FBG≤100 mg/dL (5.5mmol/L) and premixed insulin was titrated to two targets values, both a FBG≤100 mg/dL (5.5 mmol/L) and a pre-dinner BG≤100 mg/dL (5.5mmol/L), also using the "treat-to-target" weekly forced titration algorithm.

STUDY DESIGN

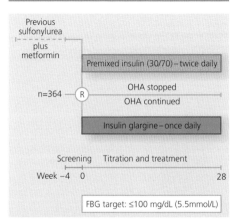

Figure 103. Design of phase IV randomized study.

OBJECTIVES

To compare the efficacy and safety of insulin glargine given once-daily in the evening combined with continued OHA to premixed insulin (30/70) monotherapy given twice daily, in insulin naïve patients with T2DM poorly controlled on their current OHAs.

BASELINE CHARACTERISTICS

	Overall population
Age (years)	61.0
BMI (kg/m²)	29.5
Duration of DM (years)	9.9
HbA_{1c} (%)	8.8
Data are means	

OUTCOME VARIABLES

- The proportion of patients reaching target HbA_{1c} ≤ 7% without documented nocturnal hypoglycemia, which was defined as BG<60 mg/dL (3.3 mmol/L)
- Baseline to endpoint changes in:
  - HbA_{1c}
  - FBG and
  - Insulin dose
  - Body weight
- 24-hour 8-point BG profile
- Documented episodes of hypoglycemia

KEY FINDINGS

- About 50% fewer patients in the premix insulin treated group reached target HbA_{1c}≤7.0 without documented nocturnal hypoglycemia (29% vs. 45%; p=0.0013)(Figure 104).
- Baseline to endpoint reductions in HbA_{1c} was significantly less with premix insulin compared to insulin glargine (–1.30% vs.–1.64%, respectively; p<0.0005).

- Insulin glargine-treated persons achieved a significantly greater reduction in FBG from baseline (-56 vs. –39 mg/dL, respectively; p<0.0001 (-3.1 vs. -2.2 mmol/L)).
- 8-point BG monitoring showed significantly better (p<0.05) glycemic control with insulin glargine at dinner, post-lunch, pre- and post-dinner and at 03.00 compared to premix.
- Patients treated with insulin glargine had significantly fewer documented hypoglycemic episodes compared to premixed insulin (mean of 1.9 vs. 4.5/patient respectively; p<0.0001)(Figure 105).
- The mean insulin dose at endpoint was higher with premix insulin (64.5 U daily)

compared to insulin glargine (28.2 U daily) (Figure 105).
- Patients treated with premix insulin experienced more weight gain (2.1 vs. 1.4 kg; respectively; p=0.08) (Figure 105).

EDITORS COMMENTARY

This study is of clinical interest in view of the widespread use of premixed insulin as monotherapy in persons with T2DM in many countries (e.g. UK, Japan, USA). A limitation of the study is that the patients randomized to treatment with premixed insulin did not continue with their OHA treatment, as was the case in the patients treated with insulin glargine. Nonetheless, the introduction of once-daily glargine at bedtime with continued OHAs restored glycemic control more effectively than PreMix, with almost one half of patients (45%) treated with insulin glargine achieving HbA$_{1c}$of ≤7.0 without any documented nocturnal hypoglycemia, which was a significantly greater number of subjects than the premix group (29%). Treatment with insulin glargine was associated with less risk of hypoglycemia, a markedly reduced insulin dose requirement and less weight gain.

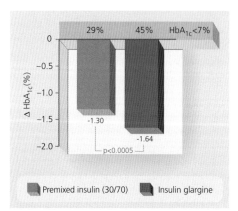

Figure 104. Baseline to endpoint change in mean HbA$_{1c}$. The proportion of patients reaching target HbA$_{1c}$ <7.0% without nocturnal hypoglycemia is shown in the shaded box.

Additional References

Janka H. Adding insulin glargine to oral hypoglycemic agents in patients with Type 2 diabetes markedly reduces insulin dose versus conventional insulin therapy. *Diabetes* 2003; 52(Supp1):A449 Abstract 1942-PO.

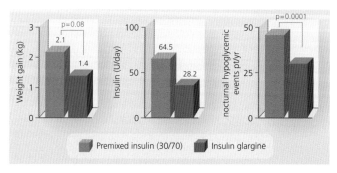

Figure 105. Findings from the study showing weight gain, insulin dose requirement and the number of nocturnal hypoglycemic events per patient-year.

Abstract

Insulin lispro mix 75/25 compared to insulin glargine in patients with type 2 diabetes new to insulin therapy.

Malone J.K, Holcombe J.H, Campaigne B.N, Kerr L.F. *Diabetes* 2004; 53(Suppl 2): Abstract 576-P.

STUDY DESCRIPTION

This randomized, open-label cross-over study comparing insulin glargine with a premixed insulin preparation was undertaken in insulin naïve persons with T2DM in multiple centers in North America. Subjects (n=105) receiving metformin were randomized to insulin glargine once-daily in the evening or twice-daily Humalog Mix 75/25 (75% NPL/25% insulin lispro) for a treatment period of 16 weeks and then crossed to the other treatment for 16 weeks.

STUDY DESIGN

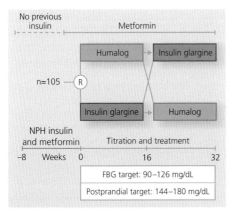

Figure 106. Design of randomized study.

BASELINE CHARACTERISTICS

	Overall population
Male (%)	63
Age (years)	55 ± 10
Duration of DM (years)	8.9 ± 6.7
Data are means ± SD	

OBJECTIVES

To compare the efficacy and safety of insulin glargine to the insulin preparation Humalog Mix 75/25 in combination with metformin in insulin naïve persons with T2DM.

OUTCOME VARIABLES

The outcome variables included:
- Baseline to endpoint change in HbA_{1C}
- The proportion of patients reaching target $HbA_{1C} \leq 7\%$
- Frequency of hypoglycemia, recorded as the rate of episodes per patient per 30 days and the proportion of patients experiencing ≥ 1 episodes
- BG, including immediate postprandial BG and 2 hour postprandial BG

KEY FINDINGS

- Significant baseline to endpoint improvements in HbA_{1C} occurred in both treatment groups (75/25: 8.6 to 7.4%, p<0.001; insulin glargine: 8.6 to 7.8%, p<0.001). Comparing the two treatment groups, there was a significantly greater reduction in mean HbA_{1C} recorded with premix 75/25 compared to insulin glargine (–1.3 ± 1.1% vs. –0.9 ± 1.1% respectively; p<0.001) and lower mean HbA_{1C} values at study endpoint were recorded with premix 75/25 compared to insulin glargine (7.4 ± 1.1% vs. 7.8 ± 1.26% respectively; p<0.001).
- A greater proportion of patients treated with 75/25 achieved target $HbA_{1C} \leq 7.0\%$ compared to insulin glargine (41.4 vs. 22.0%, respectively; p<0.001)(Figure 107).
- The increase in BG measured 2 hours after both breakfast and dinner was significantly less in persons treated with 75/25 compared to insulin glargine (after breakfast: 18 ±45 vs. 47 ± 36 mg/dL (1.0 ± 2.5 vs. 2.6 ± 2.0 mmol/L), respectively; p< 0.001 and after dinner: 14 ± 41 vs. 40 ± 40 mg/dL (0.8 ± 2.3 vs. 2.2 ± 2.2 mmol/L), respectively; p<0.001)(Figure 108).

• The overall rate of hypoglycemia was higher at study endpoint in the 75/25-treated patients compared to insulin glargine (0.68 ± 1.38 vs. 0.39 ± 1.24 episodes/patient/30 days, respectively; p=0.041), but similar rates of nocturnal hypoglycemia were recorded (0.14 ± 0.43 vs. 0.24 ± 1.10 episodes/patient /30 days, respectively; p=0.788)(Figure 109).

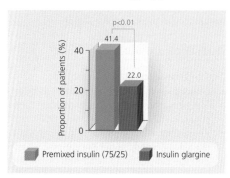

Figure 107. Proportion of patients achieving the target HbA$_{1c}$<7%.

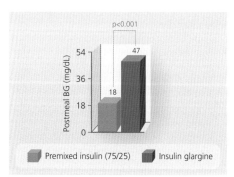

Figure 108. Increase in post breakfast (2 hour) blood glucose values.

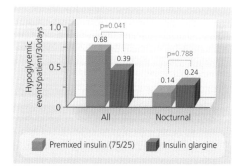

Figure 109. The number of hypoglycemic events per patient per 30-day period.

EDITORS COMMENTARY

This study underscores the importance of the insulin titration regimen and the specific FBG targets to determine the final HbA$_{1c}$ reductions. No information is provided but presumably the FBG targets for titration were higher than 100 mg/dL (5.5 mmol/L), which explains the lesser HbA$_{1c}$ reductions apparent if insulin glargine dose is not properly adjusted. Clearly, in insulin naïve patients treated with metformin, the twice-daily Humalog Mix 75/25 insulin regimen achieved a greater improvement in HbA$_{1c}$ compared to insulin glargine, which was also associated with a smaller rise in post prandial BG. These findings are reflected in the higher proportion of patients who achieved target of HbA$_{1c}$ ≤7.0% with 75/25 insulin. However, 75/25 insulin was associated with increased hypoglycemia.

The reduction of HbA$_{1c}$ of only 0.9% from a baseline of 8.6% to 7.8% with insulin glargine contrasts with other reported trials like "treat-to-target" (Riddle, Rosenstock and Gerich, 2003) and is most likely explained by the study design and the insulin titration regimen that allowed insulin glargine increments only if the FBG was >120 mg/dL. In addition, the rapid-acting insulin lispro component of the insulin mixture undoubtedly explains the lower post-prandial BG values. The second premix insulin injection in the morning especially when the FBG is > 100 mg/dL impacted on the greater HbA$_{1c}$ reductions but resulted in more overall hypoglycemia with 75/25. This study suggests that the introduction of 75/25 insulin in combination with metformin can be considered for patients with T2DM beginning insulin therapy. Despite the reductions in HbA$_{1c}$ with both insulin regimens, the proportion of patients reaching target HbA$_{1c}$ was low with insulin glargine, emphasizing the need for proper insulinization with a more aggressive and structured titration schedule so that better glycemic control can be achieved and the relative risk of hypoglycemia can be properly estimated.

Targeting postprandial rather than fasting blood glucose results in better overall glycemic control in patients with type 2 diabetes.

Abstract

Malone J.K, Bai S, Campaigne B.N, Reviriego J, Augendre-Ferrante B. *Diabetes* 2004; 53 (Suppl 2):Abstract 577P.

STUDY DESCRIPTION

This randomized, multi-center open-label 32 week crossover comparison of insulin glargine with an insulin premix preparation (Humalog Mix 75/25) was undertaken in patients with T2DM in multiple centers in North America. All subjects (n=97) were treated during a 6-week run-in period with bedtime NPH insulin plus metformin (minimum dose of 1500 mg/day) prior to randomization to twice-daily Humalog Mix 75/25 (75% NPL/25% insulin lispro) before breakfast and evening meal or insulin glargine once-daily in the evening for a treatment period of 32 weeks. During the treatment phase, both insulins were titrated to a target preprandial BG of 90 – 126 mg/dL (5 – 7 mmol/L) and in addition, 75/25 insulin was titrated to a postprandial BG of 144 – 180 mg/dL (8 – 10 mmol/L).

STUDY DESIGN

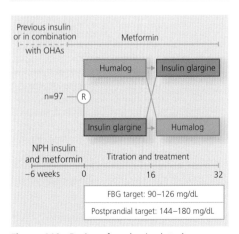

Figure 110. Design of randomized study.

OBJECTIVES

To compare glycemic response to a twice-daily insulin lispro mixture Humalog Mix 75/25 (75% NPL/25% insulin lispro) plus metformin before breakfast and evening meal or once-daily evening insulin glargine plus metformin in patients with T2DM inadequately controlled with once or twice-daily insulin alone, or in combination with OHAs.

OUTCOME VARIABLES

- Baseline to endpoint change in HbA_{1C}
- BG, including FBG and 2-hour postprandial BG
- Hypoglycemia rate (episodes/patient/30 days) and incidence (proportion of patients experiencing ≥1 episode) of overall and nocturnal hypoglycemia.

KEY FINDINGS

- A significantly lower HbA_{1C} at endpoint was achieved with 75/25 insulin compared to insulin glargine (7.54 ± 0.87% vs. 8.14 ± 1.03%, respectively; p<0.001) and this reflected a greater reduction in mean HbA_{1C} with 75/25 insulin (-1.00 vs. -0.42%, respectively; p<0.001).
- The increase in BG measured 2 hours after breakfast, lunch and dinner was significantly less (about 27 mg/dL [1.5 mmol/L]) in patients treated with 75/25 compared to insulin glargine (p< 0.001).
- Compared to the premixed 75/25 insulin, the FBG values were lower with insulin glargine (142 ± 35 vs. 133 ± 36 mg/dL (7.90 ± 1.92 vs. 7.39 ± 1.96 mmol/L) respectively; p=0.007)(Figure 111).

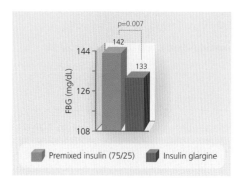

Figure 111. Fasting blood glucose at study endpoint.

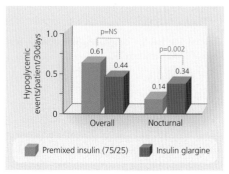

Figure 112. Frequency of hypoglycemic episodes.

- Comparing 75/25 insulin with insulin glargine, the overall rate of hypoglycemia was similar at study endpoint (0.61 ± 1.41 vs. 0.44 ± 1.07 episodes/patient/30 days, respectively; p=0.477).
- The patients treated with 75/25 insulin experienced a lower rate of nocturnal hypoglycemia compared to insulin glargine (0.14 ± 0.49 vs. 0.34 ± 0.85 episodes/patient/30 days, respectively; p=0.002).

EDITORS COMMENTARY

The study design and the specific insulin titration regimes are critical to interpret the glycemic outcomes and hypoglycemia rates in this study. In patients with T2DM inadequately controlled on once- or twice-daily insulin alone, or in combination with OHAs, a twice-daily 75/25 insulin plus metformin significantly improved HbA_{1c} and reduced nocturnal hypoglycemia, compared to once-daily insulin glargine. However, the results indicate that the insulin glargine-treated subjects were clearly under-insulinized, based on the HbA_{1c} and FBG levels described. Indeed, evening insulin adjustments were not made unless the FBG was >126 mg/dL (>7 mmol/L) which explains the high FBG of 133 mg/dL (7.39 mmol/L) and the final high HbA_{1c} of 8.1% with insulin glargine. Similarly, the FBG with 75/25 insulin was even higher at 142 mg/dL (7.90 mmol/L) which explains the lower frequency of nocturnal hypoglycemia and the lower HbA_{1c} of 7.5% was obviously achieved at the expense of the second morning injection of 75/25 insulin. Only after effective titration of the doses of insulin glargine and the 75/25 insulin can the glycemic outcomes be properly compared and then the differences in the real rate of hypoglycemia be accurately ascertained.

Comparison of intensive mixture therapy with a basal-only insulin regimen in insulin-naive patients with type 2 diabetes after failure of dual oral antihyperglycemic therapy.

Jacober SJ, Zagar AJ, Althouse SK, Pinaire JA. *Diabetes* 2004; 53(Suppl 2):Abstract 545-P.

STUDY DESCRIPTION

This randomized, open-label cross-over study enrolled insulin naïve subjects with T2DM inadequately controlled on their existing dual OHA treatment. Subjects (n=60) were randomized to one of two insulin regimens for 4 months, with cross-over to the alternative regimen for a further 4 months. The patient's OHA regimen was retained throughout the study. One of the insulin regimens involved the premixed insulin preparation consisting of Humalog Mix 50/50 before breakfast and lunch and Humalog Mix 75/25 before supper (intensive mixture therapy - IMT). The comparative regimen was insulin glargine, given once-daily at bedtime. The insulin dose was titrated to a target pre-prandial BG of <120 mg/dL (6.7 mmol/L) and 2-hour postprandial BG of <180 mg/dL (10 mmol/L), optimized without the use of a forced titration algorithm. Mean HbA_{1c} at study entry was 9.02 ± 1.24% in subjects first treated with insulin glargine and 9.40 ± 1.41% in subjects first treated with IMT.

STUDY DESIGN

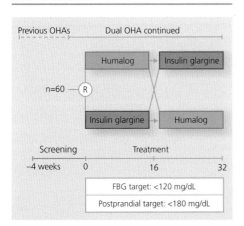

Figure 113. Design of randomized, cross-over study.

OBJECTIVES

To compare the efficacy and safety of two insulin treatment regimens, either IMT or insulin glargine, once-daily at bedtime, in poorly controlled insulin naïve patients maintaining their current OHA treatment.

OUTCOME VARIABLES

- Baseline to endpoint changes in HbA_{1c}
- The proportion of patients reaching target $HbA_{1c} \leq 7\%$
- Two-hour post-prandial and pre-dinner BG
- Documented episodes of hypoglycemia, including severe hypoglycemia

KEY FINDINGS

- The baseline to endpoint reduction in HbA_{1c} and the endpoint HbA_{1c} value were superior with IMT compared to insulin glargine (reductions of 1.08 ± 1.33% vs. -0.70 ± 1.40%, respectively (p=0.0068) and endpoint HbA_{1c} of 7.09 ± 0.74% vs. 7.33 ± 0.81%, respectively (p=0.0026)(Figure 114).
- More patients reached HbA_{1c} <7% with IMT treatment compared to insulin glargine (50 vs. 35%)(Figure 114).
- Two-hour post-prandial glucose (for all 3 meals) and pre-dinner glucose values were significantly less with IMT compared to insulin glargine (p=0.0034, p=0.0001, p=0.0066, p=0.0205, respectively).
- Hypoglycemia was twice as frequent with IMT compared to insulin glargine (4.7 ± 6.4 vs. 2.3 ± 3.2 episodes/30 days, respectively; p<0.001).
- No severe hypoglycemia was observed in either treatment group during the study.

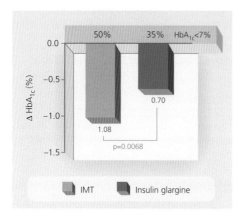

Figure 114. Mean change in HbA$_{1c}$ at study endpoint. The proportion of patients reaching target HbA$_{1c}$<7% is shown in the shaded area.

EDITORS COMMENTARY

Multiple insulin strategies can be potentially utilized to improve glycemic control when OHAs fail to maintain target HbA$_{1c}$. Basal insulin glargine in combination with OHAs is highly effective and safe but no consensus exists regarding additional alternatives such basal insulin in combination with prandial short acting analogs, premix insulin once or twice daily in combination with OHAs or a prandial multidose insulin regimen. This study compared two insulin regimens in combination with OHAs: basal insulin glargine vs. multidose prandial premix insulins.

This study was conducted in insulin naïve patients who had failed on their current dual combination OHA treatment. As expected, the intensive three-times-daily premixed insulin regimen achieved a significantly lower HbA$_{1c}$ compared to insulin glargine, with a greater proportion of patients reaching the 7% target. IMT subjects achieved lower BG values, pre- and post-prandial compared to insulin glargine, but associated with doubling of the frequency of hypoglycemia. The final HbA$_{1c}$ in a crossover study design is always difficult to interpret because of the carryover effect, but this study suggests that the introduction of three-times daily IMT can result in improved glycemic control compared to once-daily insulin glargine in insulin naïve patients continuing with dual OHA.

However, in this study, forced titration of the insulin dose was not employed and the target FBG was high at 120 mg/dL (6.7 mmol/L), which puts insulin glargine at an obvious methodological disadvantage in the control of FBG levels and subsequent daytime hyperglycemia compared to the IMT regimen, with its more aggressive prandial insulin administration irrespective of FBG levels. A more structured titration schedule to lower FBG levels, as used in the "treat-to-target" study (Riddle, Rosenstock and Gerich, 2003), could have resulted in further improvements in glycemic control with insulin glargine.

ALGORITHM COMPARISON STUDIES

AT.LANTUS trial investigating treatment algorithms for insulin glargine (Lantus®). Results of the type 2 study.

Davies M, Storms F, Shutler S, Bianchi-Biscay M, Gomis R, AT.LANTUS Study Group. *Diabetes* 2004; 53(Suppl 2):Abstract 1980–PO.

STUDY DESCRIPTION

AT.LANTUS (**A** **T**rial comparing **L**antus **A**lgorithms to achieve **N**ormal blood glucose **T**argets in subjects with **U**ncontrolled blood **S**ugar) was a randomized, open label study conducted at 611 centers in 59 countries. Persons with T2DM (4961) inadequately controlled on their current therapy (based on HbA_{1c} >7%), were randomised to two different insulin glargine dose-escalation algorithms. The first algorithm (A_1) consisted of a fixed starting dose (10 U) with titration to a FBG of 100 mg/dL (5.5 mmol/L) by 2 to 8 unit increments according to the mean FBG concentration on a weekly basis, and managed by patient practice visits. The second algorithm (A_2) had a flexible starting dose, which was determined by the initial FBG and required patient self-titration of the insulin glargine dose by increasing by 2 U every 3 days where FBG was >100 mg/dL (>5.5 mmol/L) until FBG target was achieved.

STUDY DESIGN

OBJECTIVES

To compare two "treat-to-target" algorithms for the routine clinical use of insulin glargine determined either by the health care provider or self-adjusted by the patient. The dose-escalation in each treatment algorithm was modulated by the incidence of severe hypoglycemia, which was the primary efficacy assessment in the study.

OUTCOME VARIABLES

Primary variable

• Frequency of severe hypoglycemia, defined as BG < 50 mg/dL (2.8 mmol/L) and/or needing assistance by a third person to receive oral carbohydrate or intravenous glucose or intramuscular glucagon

Secondary variables

• Frequency of nocturnal, symptomatic and asymptomatic hypoglycemia
• Baseline to endpoint changes in:
  • HbA_{1c} • Body weight
  • FBG   • Insulin dose

Mean FBG for the previous 3 consecutive days	Increase in daily basal insulin glargine dose (Units)*	
	Algorithm 1: titration at every visit	Algorithm 2: titration every 3 days
100 mg/dL and <120 mg/dL (≥5.5 mmol/L and <6.7 mmol/L)	0–2**	0–2**
120 mg/dL and <140 mg/dL (≥6.7 mmol/L and <7.8 mmol/L)	2	2
140 mg/dL and <180 mg/dL (≥7.8 mmol/L and <10 mmol/L)	4	2
≥180 mg/dL (≥10 mmol/L)	6–8**	2**

* Treat-to-target fasting blood glucose (FBG) ≤100 mg/dL (5.5 mmol/L). Titration occurred only in the absence of blood glucose levels <72 mg/dL (<4.0 mmol/L) **Magnitude of daily basal dose was at the discretion of the investigator.

Table 10. Comparison of adjustments in the daily basal insulin glargine dose between the two treatment algorithms.

KEY FINDINGS

- Both insulin titration regimens were safe with low frequency of severe hypoglycemia.
- There was no significant difference between the two treatment algorithms (A_1 and A_2) in the frequency of severe hypoglycemia (0.9 vs. 1.1%, respectively).
- Comparing treatment algorithms A_1 and A_2, significantly fewer nocturnal (3.2 vs. 4.1%) and symptomatic (26.3 vs. 29.7%) hypoglycemic events were apparent with A_1, with no difference in the frequency of asymptomatic hypoglycemia.
- In both treatment arms, subjects experienced significant baseline to endpoint decreases in HbA_{1c} (mean reduction from 8.98 to 7.78% p<0.001). Comparing treatment algorithms A_1 and A_2, subjects achieved a significantly lower HbA_{1c} with A_2 (-1.08 vs. -1.22%, p<0.001).
- In both treatment arms, patients experienced a significant baseline to endpoint decrease in FBG (mean reduction from 169.6 to 110.3 mg/dL (9.4 to 6.1 mmol/L), p<0.001). A significantly larger mean reduction in FBG was achieved with A_2 (-56.9 vs. -61.7 mg/dL (3.2 vs. 3.4 mmol/L), p<0.001).
- The final basal insulin dose recorded was overall very low but slightly higher with A_2 (A_1 vs. A_2: 0.12 vs. 0.15 U/kg, p=0.02).
- There was no difference in weight gain between the two algorithms.

Additional References

1. Davies M and Jarvis J. A trial comparing Lantus algorithms to achieve normal blood glucose targets in type 2 diabetes subjects with uncontrolled blood sugar. *Diabetes* 2003; 52 (Suppl 1): Abstract 1928-PO.

EDITORS COMMENTARY

Translational studies are important to assess how novel therapeutic strategies can be applied from the research arena into the global clinical environment. Specifically, the basal insulin glargine titration strategy using the "treat-to-target" doses under health care provider supervision needed to be tested against an even simpler insulin titration regimen that could empower the patient to self-adjust consistently utilizing on lower insulin doses.

The findings of this study demonstrate the benefits of both a physician-driven and a patient-self managed algorithm in improving glycemic control in persons with poorly controlled T2DM. The study results show that the simpler patient-self managed algorithm achieved better glycemic control with very little difference between the algorithms with respect to frequency of hypoglycemia. This is encouraging and supports the view that empowering the patient to effectively self-adjust is a critical feature in achieving good glycemic control. The reductions of HbA_{1c} in the range of 1.1-1.2% were obtained with very low insulin glargine doses of < 0.2 units/kg which suggests that even greater HbA_{1c} reductions could have been achieved if the titration regimen was consistently followed. It is also important to note that 72% of patients were already receiving insulin at baseline, with a mean diabetes duration of 12.3 years. This may also explain why, in this advanced diabetes population, HbA_{1c} of 7% was not reached. Looking to the future, this study supports the view that patient education involving the setting of FBG targets and the self-titration of insulin glargine dose may be a viable strategy to empower and engage further the person with T2DM in an attempt to further improve glycemic control.

Effect of basal insulin glargine therapy in type 2 patients inadequately controlled on oral antidiabetic agents: AT.LANTUS trial results.

Lavalle-González F, Storms F, Shutler S, Bianchi-Biscay M, Gomis R, Davies M, AT.LANTUS Study Group. *Diabetes* 2004; 53(Suppl 2):Abstract 12-LB.

Abstract

STUDY DESCRIPTION

This was an additional analysis of the AT.LANTUS study (**A** **T**rial comparing **L**antus **A**lgorithms to achieve **N**ormal blood glucose **T**argets in subjects with **U**ncontrolled blood **S**ugar). This analysis was undertaken to examine the glycemic control achieved in the subgroup of subjects enrolled into the study who were poorly controlled on >1 OHA (n=962; 19.4% of randomized patients). Subjects who received insulin glargine with one oral agent (n=340) or more than one agent (n=525) had been randomized to two different insulin glargine dose-escalation algorithms. The first algorithm (A_1) consisted of a fixed starting dose (10 U) with titration to a FBG of 100 mg/dL (5.5 mmol/L) by 2 to 8 unit increments according to the mean FBG concentration on a weekly basis, and managed by patient practice visits. The second algorithm (A_2) had a flexible starting dose, which was determined by the initial FBG and required patient self-titration of the insulin glargine dose by increasing by 2 U every 3 days where FBG was >100 mg/dL (>5.5 mmol/L) until FBG target was achieved.

OBJECTIVE

The aim of this AT.LANTUS sub-analysis was to compare two different "treat-to-target" algorithms for the routine clinical use of insulin glargine either determined by the health care provider or self-adjusted by the patient in the subgroup of T2DM subjects inadequately controlled on OHAs. The dose-escalation in each treatment algorithm was modulated by the incidence of severe hypoglycemia, which was the primary efficacy assessment in the study.

OUTCOME VARIABLES

- Frequency of severe hypoglycemia (BG < 50 mg/dL (2.8 mmol/L) and /or needing assistance by a third person to receive oral carbohydrate or intravenous glucose or intramuscular glucagons), symptomatic and nocturnal hypoglycemia
- Overall glycemic control assessed by HbA_{1c} and FBG concentrations
- Baseline to endpoint change in:
  - Insulin dose
  - Body weight

KEY FINDINGS

- There were significant decreases in HbA_{1c} and FBG in all patients (Table 11).
- Comparing treatment algorithm A_1 to A_2, the endpoint HbA_{1c} was significantly lower with A_2 both in patients treated with a single OHA (7.9% vs. 7.5%, p=0.03) and multiple OHA (7.6% vs. 7.3%, p<0.005).
- Endpoint FBG was also significantly lower with A_2 both in patients treated with a single OHA (FBG: 117 vs. 107 mg/dL, p<0.005) and multiple OHA (114 vs. 104 mg/dL, p<0.005).
- More patients achieved target HbA_{1c} of 7% with A_2 (42.7% vs. 31.1%).
- The final insulin dose was significantly higher (p<0.001) with A_2 in both groups (Table 11).
- Overall, there was a low incidence of severe hypoglycemia (<1%).

		Insulin glargine + single OHA		Insulin glargine + multiple OHA	
		A₁	A₂	A₁	A₂
HBA₁c	Baseline	9.1 ± 1.3	9.1 ± 1.3	9.1 ± 1.3	9.2 ± 1.2
	End	7.9 ± 1.1	7.5 ± 1.2*	7.6 ± 1.2	7.3 ± 1.0**
FBG (mg/dL)	Baseline	180.7 ± 45.8	186.2 ± 55.3	180.4 ± 46.5	183.7 ± 47.8
	End	117.2 ± 31.6	107.2 ± 27.2**	113.9 ± 27.4	104.1 ± 23.2***
Insulin dose (U)	Baseline	10.0 ± 0.4	12.2 ± 4.4	10.2 ± 1.3	11.6 ± 3.1
	End	37.4 ± 19.1***	46.1 ± 26.6***	30.1 ± 15.3***	34.5 ± 22.2***

*p=0.03; **p=0.001; ***p<0.001

Table 11. Summary of findings in AT.LANTUS findings in the subgroup of insulin naïve patients inadequately controlled on OHA treatment alone.

EDITORS COMMENTARY

Study design and consistent insulin titration to specific FBG target <100 mg/dL remain the most critical factors to achieve substantial HbA₁c reductions. This additional analysis of a subgroup of subjects in the AT.LANTUS study shows that patients poorly controlled on their current OHAs can effectively reduce their FBG and HbA₁c, with about 30 - 40 % achieving glycemic target HbA₁c of 7% using either of the treatment algorithms investigated, with few episodes of hypoglycemia. These data clearly show that the subjects adopting self-titration of their insulin glargine using a simple algorithm of a 2 U increase every three days based on self-measured FBG more effectively reached target glycemic control. These patients also achieved the largest fall in FBG, reflecting the substantially higher doses of insulin used at study endpoint, in particular in the patients switched to insulin glargine with one oral agent. As expected better HbA₁c reductions with lower insulin requirements were obtained in patients on combination OHAs with insulin glargine as compared with those receiving only a single OHA with insulin glargine. These findings mirror the results of the complete cohort and show that patients can effectively participate in managing their own insulin dose by self adjustment to achieve >1.8% absolute reduction in HbA₁c.

Treat-to-target simply – the LANMET study.

Yki-Järvinen H, Hänninen J, Hulme S, Kauppinen-Mäkelin R, Lahdenperä S, Lehtonen R, Levanen H, Nikkiä K, Ryysy L, Tiikkainen M, Tulokas T, Virtamo H, Vahatalo M.

Diabetes 2004; 53(Suppl 2):Abstract 2181-PO.

Abstract

STUDY DESCRIPTION

This open label study, conducted at multiple centers in Europe, randomized 110 insulin-naive patients with poorly controlled T2DM (mean HbA$_{1c}$ of 9.5 ± 0.1%) to treatment with 2000 mg metformin daily and once daily bedtime insulin therapy, either NPH insulin or insulin glargine for a period of 9 months. Patients were instructed to increase their daily insulin dose by 2 U every 3 days if their FPG was above the target range of 72–100 mg/dL (4.0 - 5.6 mmol/L). The dose escalation was halted by the occurrence of hypoglycemic episodes. The dose escalation was monitored at a diabetes treatment center by reviewing FPG values transferred into the center by modem, in conjunction with less frequent (3-monthly) physician contact.

OBJECTIVES

To compare the efficacy of bedtime NPH insulin and insulin glargine in achieving target glycemic control with patient self-adjustment of insulin dose using a very simple titration regimen in insulin naïve patients with inadequate glycemic control.

KEY FINDINGS

- FPG was reduced to average values of 103 ± 1 mg/dL (5.7 ± 0.1 mmol/L) with insulin glargine treatment and 108 ± 1 mg/dL (6 ± 0.1 mmol/L) with NPH insulin.
- The insulin dose recorded at study endpoint was similar in each treatment arm: 68 ± 5 with insulin glargine and 70 ± 6 U with NPH insulin, with insulin doses ranging from 20 – 194 U (Figure 115a).
- The mean HbA$_{1c}$ was reduced from 9.5 ± 0.1% to 7.1 ± 0.1% in both treatment groups.
- Symptomatic hypoglycemia occurred significantly more frequently (44% higher) with NPH insulin compared to insulin glargine (8.0 vs. 5.5 episodes/patient-year, respectively; p<0.05)(Figure 115b).
- During the day, the mean PG values recorded were higher with NPH insulin compared to insulin glargine, both before (182 ± 5 vs. 155 ± 5 mg/dL; p=0.002) and after evening meal (221 ± 5 vs. 202 ± 5 mg/dL; p<0.03).
- Average weight gain tended to be higher in the NPH insulin patients compared to insulin glargine-treated patients, but this was not significant (3.5 ± 0.7 vs. 2.6 ± 0.6 kg, respectively; p=NS) (Figure 115c).

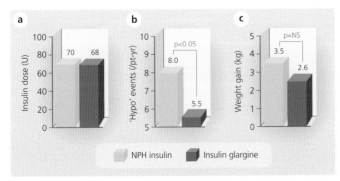

Figure 115. (a) Insulin dose at study endpoint. (b) Frequency of symptomatic hypoglycemic episodes, expressed as events per patient-year. (c) Weight gain experienced during the 9 month study.

EDITORS COMMENTARY

The LANMET study set out to determine if good glycemic control could be achieved by patients self-adjusting their insulin dose according to their self monitored FPG levels based on a very simple predefined algorithm. The home plasma glucose levels were transmitted to the diabetes treatment center using a modem. The insulin dose adjustment algorithm required infrequent, 3-monthly physician contact.

Effective glycemic control was restored, with the mean HbA$_{1c}$ almost to target level, and as expected, in the case of NPH insulin this was achieved at the cost of a much higher frequency of hypoglycemic events, and consequently a tendency to greater weight gain compared to insulin glargine. The insulin dose escalation achieved in this way was very effective. These findings extend those of other previous insulin dose algorithm-based studies. The "treat-to-target" study (Rosenstock et al., 2003) showed that adopting a forced titration algorithm of insulin dose effectively improved glycemic control, with fewer hypoglycemic episodes occurring in patients treated with insulin glargine compared to NPH insulin. The AT.LANTUS study showed that a similar, simple patient self-titration schedule was probably more effective than the more complex physician-driven algorithm for improving glycemic control. From this LANMET study, we conclude that good glycemic control can be achieved with a simple basal insulin dose titration regimen plus metformin requiring less frequent physician contact. In this context, insulin glargine was associated with markedly improved HbA$_{1c}$ less hypoglycemia, better pre- and post-dinner glucose control and slightly less weight gain compared to NPH insulin.

OBSERVATIONAL STUDIES

Metabolic and weight benefits following long-term administration of insulin glargine (Lantus®) in patients with type 2 diabetes in clinical practice.

Schreiber S, Rußmann A. *Diabetes Metabolism* 2003; 29(Spec No 2):Abstract 2212.

STUDY DESCRIPTION

This was a single center, long-term observational study. The findings described in several abstracts have been combined and summarized. Patients (mean age 60.2 years, mean body weight 94.9 kg) receiving treatment with OHA only (n=16), OHA plus insulin (n=11), conventional insulin therapy (CIT)(n=10) or intensified conventional insulin therapy (ICT) (n=23) were switched to receive insulin glargine once-daily in conjunction with continued OHA and/or prandial insulin for 18 months. Patients were enrolled based on either inadequate glycemic control (FBG>140mg/dL), or on the basis that their previous insulin treatment regimen was considered by the patient to be too rigid. Patients either took part in a formal educational program on insulin and diet at baseline and/or underwent routine physician consultations throughout the course of this study.

OBJECTIVES

To determine the long-term efficacy and safety of insulin glargine in a clinical practice in persons with T2DM who were poorly controlled or dissatisfied on their current treatment regimen.

OUTCOME VARIABLES

Primary variables
- Changes in the HbA_{1c} level from baseline at 9 and 18 months
- Changes in body weight from baseline at 9 and 18 months

Secondary variables
- Patient reported episodes of severe hypoglycemia

KEY FINDINGS

- Overall, patients switched to treatment with insulin glargine experienced a significant decrease from baseline in HbA_{1c} at 9 months (reduction from 8.1 to 7.3%, p<0.001) and 18 months (reduction from 8.1% to 6.9%, (p<0.0003) (Figure 116).
- Patients previously treated with insulin as ICT or CIT showed no change in glycemic control. With ICT, the HbA_{1c} was 6.0, 7.1 and 6.7 % at baseline, 9 and 18 months respectively. With CIT, the HbA_{1c} was 7.0, 7.0 and 6.9 % at baseline, 9 and 18 months respectively (Figure 116).
- Patients who had previously received OHA monotherapy achieved a significant reduction in HbA_{1c} at 9 months (-1.4%; p<0.05) to 7% and was maintained at 18 months (Figure 116).
- Patients who had previously received OHA in conjunction with insulin also achieved significant reductions in HbA_{1c} at 9 months (-2.1%; p<0.05) to 7.2% and was maintained at 18 months (Figure116).
- For all patients, the mean weight loss at 9 and 18 months was 1.1kg and 8.2 kg respectively (Figure 117).
- In patients previously treated with ICT, there was a mean weight loss of 1.5 kg and 14 kg at 9 and 18 months respectively. With CIT, the mean weight loss was 0.3kg at 9 months and 7.7 kg at 18 months (Figure 117).
- In patients pre-treated with OHA with or without insulin, there was minimal weight change over the 18 months study period (Figure 117).
- No episodes of severe hypoglycemia were reported by the patients during the study period.

Abstract

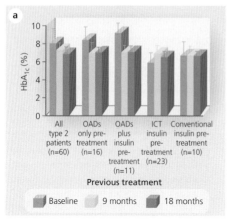

Figure 116. Baseline to endpoint changes in HbA$_{1c}$.

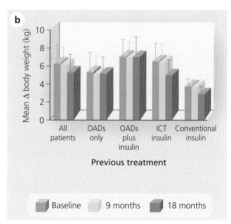

Figure 117. Baseline to endpoint changes in body weight.

EDITORS COMMENTARY

In this long-term study, insulin glargine treatment in association with an "insulin and diet" education program was successful in achieving and/or maintaining good glycemic control in patients previously treated either with OHA alone, or with insulin, as a conventional treatment (CIT) or as intensified conventional therapy (ICT). Both the improvement in glycemic control and the significant weight loss recorded reflect the expertise of a specialized diabetes center, with an emphasis on dietary and lifestyle intervention.

Those patients on OHA alone or OHA in conjunction with insulin had a reduction in HbA$_{1c}$ of 1.4% and 1.1%, with end-of-treatment means of HbA$_{1c}$ of 7% and 7.2%, respectively, and accompanied by a 1.4 kg and 1.0 kg change in body weight over 18 months. In patients who had previously received insulin as CIT or as ICT, HbA$_{1c}$ was maintained at below 7% in both groups at 18 months. In these groups, a significant weight loss was observed. Weight loss has always been very difficult to accomplish in clinical practice. In the absence of a control group, no definitive conclusions can be strongly stated. Nonetheless, insulin glargine appeared to be an effective tool to facilitate implementation of glycemic control and weight loss in a structured diabetes program, presumably due to the reckless profile and reduced risk of hypoglycemia without the need for supplemented caloric intake.

This study confirms the efficacy of insulin glargine as a basal insulin supplement in a "real world" clinical setting. Insulin glargine therefore offers patients under intensive insulin therapy a less rigid and equally effective insulin treatment regimen.

Additional References

1. Schreiber S, Rußmann A. Long-term administration of insulin glargine (LANTUS®): Metabolic and weight benefits in patients with type 2 diabetes in clinical practice. *Diabetes* 2003; 52(Suppl 1):A455 Abstract 1972.

2. Schreiber S, Rußman A. Improved metabolic control with a favourable weight profile in patients with type 2 diabetes treated with insulin glargine in clinical practice. *Diabetes* 2002; 51(Suppl 1):A114 Abstract 464-P.

3. Schreiber S, Rußman A. Improved metabolic control in patients with type 1 and type 2 diabetes following the initiation/switching to insulin glargine in clinical practice. *Diabetes* 2002; 51(Suppl 1):A114 Abstract 465-P.

Treatment with insulin glargine of patients with type 2 diabetes in clinical practice: metabolic control over 30 months.

Schreiber S, Russmann A. *Diabetes* 2004; 53(Suppl 2):Abstract 2043-PO.

STUDY DESCRIPTION

This is an additional analysis of a single center, long-term observational study assessing patients with T2DM treated with insulin glargine. This particular analysis was conducted on a group of patients (n=46) with near-normal weight (mean body weight 86.3 ± 17.7 kg) who failed on their current therapy of OHA or insulin and then were given insulin glargine, once-daily, for 30 months in clinical practice. As previously described, patients were enrolled based on either inadequate glycemic control with FBG>140mg/dL (7.8 mmol/L), or on the basis that their previous insulin treatment regimen was regarded by the patient to be too rigid. In this analysis, the patients were investigated according to their previous treatment, with OHAs (n=18) or insulin only (n=28). Subjects' metabolic control was assessed at 9, 18, 24 and 30 months. The dose of insulin glargine was titrated according to the morning FBG. Subjects involved in the study either took part in a formal educational program on insulin and diet at baseline and/or underwent routine physician consultations during the course of this study.

KEY FINDINGS

- Significant reductions from baseline HbA_{1c} (8.14% ± 1.7%) were observed at 9 and 30 months in all the patients (reductions from baseline of -0.69% (p<0.002) and -0.96%, respectively (p<0.001)) (Table 12; Figure 118).
- The patients treated previously with OHAs experienced greater reductions from a higher baseline HbA_{1c} of 9.16% ± 1.7% [-1.88% at 9 months (p<0.002) and -2.26 % at 30 months (p<0.001)] (Table 12; Figure 118).
- The insulin-only pre-treated group experienced smaller but significant reductions from a baseline of 7.59 ± 1.5% (-0.09% at 9 months (p<0.001) and 0.38% at 30 months (p<0.001) (Table 12; Figure 118).
- There was no change in weight from baseline to endpoint.
- No unexpected adverse events or episodes of severe hypoglycemia were observed.

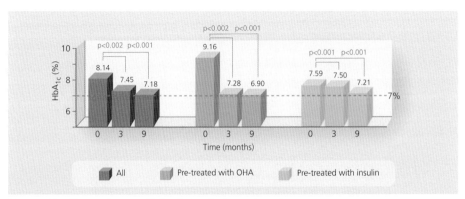

Figure 118. Changes in mean HbA_{1c} during the 9 month study

	All patients	Previous OHA	Previous insulin only
Baseline	8.14 ± 1.7	9.16 ± 1.7	7.59 ± 1.5
9 months	7.45 ± 0.9	7.28 ± 1.0	7.50 ± 1.0
Δ at 9 months	−0.69 (p<0.002)	−1.88 (p<0.002)	−0.09 (p<0.001)
30 months	7.18 ± 0.9	6.90 ± 0.3	7.21 ± 1.1
Δ at 30 months	−0.96 (p<0.001)	−2.26 (p<0.001)	−0.38 (p<0.001)

Table 12. Summary of the findings of the 30 month observational study. Difference (Δ) and p values are shown.

EDITORS COMMENTARY

This uncontrolled study has clear limitations, but provides some valuable long term observations indicating sustained glycemic effects and no weight gain when insulin glargine is part of an integrated diabetes management program in clinical practice. In combination with educational support, the addition of insulin glargine to persons inadequately controlled or dissatisfied with their current insulin therapy significantly improved their glycemic control over a period of 30 months.

As expected, the greatest reduction in HbA_{1c} was seen in those subjects previously treated with OHA alone, with a mean value less than target at 30 months. It is important to note that none of the subjects were recorded as having experienced unexpected adverse events, episodes of severe hypoglycemia and no weight gain was evident in these patients who entered this long-term study with near-normal body weight.

Twelve-month effectiveness of insulin glargine use in diabetic patients from an endocrinology speciality practice.

Fischer J, Roberts C, McLaughlin T, Loza L, Beauchamp R, Antell L, Schwartz S, Kipnes M.
Diabetes 2003; 52(Suppl 1):A446 Abstract 1933-PO

Abstract

STUDY DESCRIPTION

This large, long-term single center, retrospective, observational study described treatment with insulin glargine in persons with either T1DM (Group A, findings not included below) or T2DM. Those patients on insulin alone or insulin plus OHA had their bedtime NPH insulin substituted by insulin glargine (Group B). Insulin naïve patients receiving OHA only were initiated on bedtime insulin glargine whilst continuing OHAs (Group C). Outcome variables were described at 6 months (n=445) and reported separately as Group B (n=390) and Group C (n=55) patients. In a separate report of the same study, combined data (Groups B and C combined; n=180) at baseline and 12 months were reported. The outcome measures included QoL at 12 months (n=36).

OBJECTIVES

To assess impact of the introduction of insulin glargine on glycemic control and weight (BMI) in persons with T2DM previously treated with either bedtime NPH insulin or only OHAs.

OUTCOME VARIABLES

- Changes from baseline to 6 months and 12 months in:
  - HbA_{1c}
  - BMI
  - Hypoglycemic episodes (at 12 months only)
- QoL measures at 0, 2, 6, 12 and 16 weeks post-therapy initiation.

KEY FINDINGS

- A significant reduction in HbA_{1c} levels from baseline occurred at 6 months and 12 months (Figure 119):
  - Group B patients at 6 months (-0.71 ± 1.77%; p<0.0001).
  - Group C patients at 6 months (-1.58 ± 1.56%; p<0.0001).
  - Group B+C at 12 months (-0.60 ± 1.51%; p<0.001).

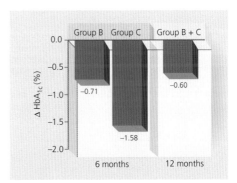

Figure 119. Change in HbA_{1c} during study period.

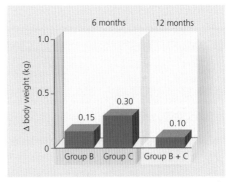

Figure 120. Weight change during study period.

- The improvement in glycemic control did not result in a significant change from baseline in BMI, either in the Group B and C patients at 6 months or the combined Group B+C at 12 months, following the introduction of insulin glargine (Figure 120).
- There were fewer hypoglycemic events per patient in the year following the introduction of insulin glargine compared to the pre-study year in the combined Groups B+C (p=0.004).
- Standardized assessments of QoL, that is overall and emotional well being, total symptom score and total symptom distress score, were all significantly improved with insulin glargine therapy.

EDITORS COMMENTARY

This uncontrolled "real world" collection of data on the effect of insulin glargine introduction revealed significant improvements in glycemic control in all treatment groups at 6 months, especially the insulin-naïve patients, and with no clinically meaningful weight gain. Similarly, a significant reduction in HbA$_{1c}$ with little or no weight gain was seen in those patients monitored over a 12 month period. In a subpopulation in which QoL measures were recorded, after 4 months positive changes were seen in favor of the introduction of insulin glargine.

Additional References

1. Fischer JS, Dirani RG, Schwartz SL, Kipnes MS, Trigoso FW, Salhin AA, Vadakekalam J, Dreimane D, Loza L. Impact of use of insulin glargine on HbA$_{1c}$ and BMI in a specialty (endocrine) practice population. *Diabetes* 2002; 51(Suppl 1):A97 Abstract 393-P

Treatment of patients with type 2 diabetes with insulin glargine in everyday clinical practice.

Klinge A, Schneider K, Schweitzer MA. *Diabetes Metabolism* 2003; 29(Spec No 2): Abstract 2208.

Abstract

STUDY DESCRIPTION

This open-label, multicenter observational study of 3 months duration was undertaken in 7182 patients by 1345 physicians. All patients were inadequately controlled on their current therapy, either with OHAs (79.6%), or insulin (23.2%). Patients received once-daily insulin glargine and continued with OHA therapy. Those on insulin therapy stopped their previous regimen and switched to insulin glargine with OHA. Decisions regarding treatment and dosing were made at the discretion of the attending physicians, based on individual blood glucose levels and reflecting clinical practice in Germany.

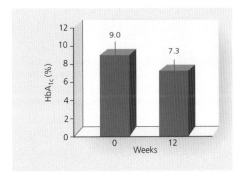

Figure 121. Three month findings of HbA_{1c}. Error bars shown are standard deviations.

OBJECTIVES

To investigate metabolic control in persons with T2DM initiated on insulin glargine as the basal insulin in the setting of everyday clinical practice.

OUTCOME VARIABLES

- Changes from baseline to 2, 4, 8 and 12 weeks in:
  - HbA_{1c}
  - FBG
  - Pre-lunch and pre-dinner BG
  - Insulin dose
  - BMI (week 12 only)

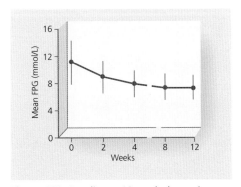

Figure 122. Baseline to 12-week change in mean fasting blood glucose.

KEY FINDINGS

- Mean HbA_{1c} decreased from 9.0 ± 2.0% at baseline to 7.3±1.3% at 3 months (Figure 121).
- Mean FBG reduced from 200 ± 56 mg/dL (11.0 ± 3.1 mmol/L) at baseline to 120 ± 27 mg/dL (6.9 ± 1.5 mmol/L) (Figure 122).
- Mean BG measured before lunch decreased from 200 ± 60 mg/dL (11.1 ± 3.3 mmol/L) at base line to 133 ± 31 mg/dL (7.3 ± 1.7 mmol/L) at 3 months and before dinner decreased from 200 ± 58 mg/dL (11.0 ± 3.2 mmol/L) to 133 ± 31 mg/dL (7.4 ± 1.7 mmol/L) at the study endpoint.
- The mean initial dose of insulin glargine was 14.3 U/day at baseline and increased to 19.7 U/day by the end of the study.
- Mean body weight and BMI remained unchanged over the course of the study.

EDITORS COMMENTARY

The findings of this large, observational study extend those obtained under the controlled conditions of clinical trials to the setting of everyday clinical practice. Persons with T2DM inadequately controlled by OHA benefited from the initiation of basal insulin therapy with insulin glargine. After 12 weeks of treatment with a low daily dose of insulin glargine (about 20 units), HbA_{1c} levels were substantially lowered, almost to target levels of <7%, and diurnal and fasting blood glucose were improved. This improvement in metabolic control was achieved without weight gain. The lack of weight gain is noteworthy, and probably reflects a reduced frequency of hypoglycemia. Traditionally, one should state that these results need to be interpreted with caution due to the lack of a control group. However, the purpose of the study was to assess the translational value and the impact of the insulin glargine/OHA regimen in clinical practice in Germany.

Basal insulin supplement in type 2 diabetic patients treated by intensified insulin therapy (IIT): glargine vs. NPH insulin.

Jungmann E, Mertens C, Snelting U, Jungmann G. *European Journal of Clinical Investigation* 2001; 31(Suppl 1):11 Abstract 46.

Abstract

STUDY DESCRIPTION

This single center, non-randomized comparison study enrolled 143 persons with T2DM who were being initiated onto insulin therapy. The patients received basal insulin supplementation, either insulin glargine given at bedtime (n=46) or NPH insulin once- or twice-daily (n=97).

OBJECTIVES

To compare the efficacy and acceptability of a single bedtime dose evening dose of insulin glargine compared to once- or twice-daily NPH insulin in an in-patient treatment program for the initiation of an intensified insulin therapy program.

OUTCOME VARIABLES

- FBG
- Severe hypoglycemia
- Insulin dosage
- Patient well-being
- Adverse events

KEY FINDINGS

- There was a significantly higher FBG recorded at 08.00 with NPH insulin compared to insulin glargine (155 ± 4 mg/dL vs.139 ± 5 mg/dL; p<0.05)(Figure 123).
- There were no significant symptomatic hypoglycemic events recorded.
- The daily dosage of NPH insulin and insulin glargine was similar (Figure 124).
- The use of concomitant metformin therapy was significantly higher in the NPH insulin-treated patients compared to

insulin glargine-treated patients (25% vs. 9%; p<0.05).
- There were no study drop-outs for other reasons.

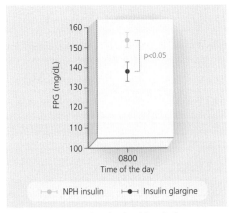

Figure 123. Morning fasting blood glucose levels.

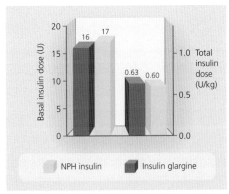

Figure 124. Insulin glargine dose and total insulin dose.

EDITORS COMMENTARY

This single practice study comparing once- or twice-daily NPH insulin to once-daily insulin glargine has only been described in abstract form and therefore the information presented is limited. It is unclear how the patients were chosen for each insulin and how the insulin doses were adjusted. Clearly the patients received basal/bolus insulin therapy but no data are described on the prandial insulin regimen used.

The data shows that insulin glargine was associated with lower levels of FBG in the morning at equivalent doses. No severe hypoglycemia was noted in either treatment group. Interestingly, fewer patients treated with insulin glargine received concomitant metformin treatment.

Additional References

1. Jungmann E, Mertens C, Snelting U, Jungmann G. Basal insulin supplement in type 2 diabetic patients treated by intensified insulin therapy (IIT): glargine vs. NPH Insulin. *Diabetes Stoffwechsel* 2001: 10(Suppl 1):70 Abstract 10-28.

Combined insulin glargine and metformin therapy for obese patients with type 2 diabetes mellitus.

Stryjek-Kaminska D, Plininger I, Jaursch-Hancke C. *Diabetes* 2002; 51(Suppl 2): A423 Abstract 2531-P.

STUDY DESCRIPTION

This single center observational study enrolled 42 persons with T2DM in whom dietary measures and OHA had failed to achieve adequate glycemic control (mean BMI 33.2 kg/m^2, FBG>155 mg/dL and HbA$_{1c}$ >8.5%). All patients were treated with once-daily insulin glargine plus metformin over a 12-week period.

OBJECTIVES

To describe the efficacy and safety of an evening dose of insulin glargine combined with twice-daily metformin (850 mg) over a 12-week period in persons with T2DM who were inadequately controlled on their current OHA treatment.

OUTCOME VARIABLES

- Baseline to endpoint changes in:
  - FBG
  - HbA$_{1c}$
  - Body weight
  - Total cholesterol and triglyceride levels
- Hypoglycemic episodes, defined as BG<50mg/dL (2.5 mmol/L).
- Adverse events

KEY FINDINGS

- Comparing baseline to endpoint, FBG was significantly reduced (mean (± SD): 206 ± 46 (11.4 ± 2.6 mmol/L) vs. 105 ± 32 mg/dL (5.8 ± 1.8 mmol/L); p<0.001).
- Comparing baseline to endpoint, HbA$_{1c}$ was significantly reduced: 9.8 ± 1.3% vs. 8.2 ± 0.9%; p<0.001).
- No hypoglycemic events were recorded.
- Patient body weight remained essentially unchanged during the study (mean change 0.2 ± 1.6 kg).

- Comparing baseline to endpoint, serum total cholesterol (217 to 191 mg/dL, p<0.05) and serum total triglyceride levels (238 to 207 mg/dL, p<0.03) were significantly reduced.
- In the first week, six patients reported mild side effects thought to be associated with the introduction of metformin therapy (diarrhea, abdominal discomfort). This did not result in any patients withdrawing from the study.

EDITORS COMMENTARY

This is a small observational study in which insulin glargine was introduced together with metformin in obese persons with T2DM. Over a 12-week period, patients showed significantly improved metabolic control, including improvement of total cholesterol and triglyceride levels, with no weight gain. There were no severe hypoglycemic events described in any patient.

The HbA$_{1c}$ reduction of 1.6% was significant after 12 weeks but it still remained at an unacceptable level, above the target of 7%. It is interesting that the FBG was markedly reduced to close to 100 mg/dL, but the final HbA$_{1c}$ was around 8%, which could be explained by the markedly elevated levels at study entry suggesting more advanced T2DM that would necessitate postprandial glucose control with the addition of short acting analogs. Alternatively, it is conceivable that use of a secretagog could have enhanced any remaining endogenous insulin secretion. These explanations are only hypothetical, but can be investigated with properly designed controlled studies.

Abstract

Insulin glargine in type 2 diabetes: An observational study of everyday practice.

Schreiber S.A, Schneider K, Schweitzer MA. *Diabetes* 2004; 53(Suppl 2):Abstract 2043-PO.

STUDY DESCRIPTION

This 9-month, uncontrolled study, is the largest observational trial (n=12,216) reported. The study enrolled patients with T2DM inadequately controlled on their current OADs to assess the effect of add-on insulin glargine treatment. This was a "real world" study conducted in the setting of general clinical practice without any strict rigorous protocol. Decisions regarding insulin glargine dosing including changes on OAD treatment were made at the discretion of the attending physician and reflecting everyday practice. Almost half the patients (47%) had T2DM for more than 5 years duration and 39% of the patients had T2DM for 1-5 years. Interestingly, 10% of the patients had T2DM for <1 year and the remaining 4% were recently diagnosed.

OBJECTIVES

The aim of this observational study was to investigate the effect of adding insulin glargine basal therapy to OHAs in patients with T2DM in the setting of everyday practice.

OUTCOME VARIABLES

- Baseline, 3-month and 9-month changes in:
  - HbA_{1c}
  - FBG
  - Insulin dose
  - Body weight and BMI
- Adverse drug reactions, including hypoglycemia

KEY FINDINGS

- After 3 months of treatment, reductions in HbA_{1c} were apparent (8.7 ± 1.4% reduced to 7.2 ± 0.9%) and this was maintained at 9 months (7.0 ± 1.0%)(Table 13; Figure 125a).
- FBG was substantially reduced from baseline levels (202 ± 56 mg/dL, 11.2 ± 3.1 mmol/L) at 3 months (133 ± 32 mg/dL, 7.4 ± 1.8 mmol/L) with little additional reduction at 9 months (131 ± 34 mg/dL, 7.3 ± 1.9 mmol/L)(Table 13; Figure 125b).
- No weight gain occurred with the addition of insulin glargine. BMI was reduced slightly from 29.0 ± 4.7 to 28.7 ± 4.5 kg/m^2

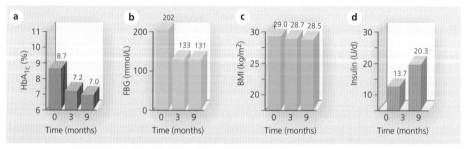

Figure 125. Summary of main findings during 9 month study period (**a**) Change in mean HbA_{1c} (**b**) Change in mean fasting blood glucose (**c**) Change in mean BMI (**d**) Increase in mean insulin dose.

during the 3-month treatment period (Table 13; Figure 125c).

- BMI was reduced slightly to 28.5 ± 4.8 kg/m^2 during the 9-month treatment period (Table 13; Figure 125c).

- The mean starting dose of insulin glargine (13.7 ± 7.0 U) increased to 20.3 ± 9.6 U at 9 months (Figure 125d).

- Adverse drug reactions were documented in 26 patients (0.21%). Only 19 of 47 adverse events documented were due to hypoglycemia.

	HbA$_{1c}$ (%)	FBG (mg/dL)	BMI (kg/m^2)
Baseline	8.7 ±1.4 (n=11,511)	202 ± 56 (n=12,100)	29.0 ± 4.7 (n=11,090)
3 months	7.2 ±0.9 (n=11,296)	133 ± 32 (n=11,872)	28.7 ± 4.5 (n=10,692)
9 months	7.0 ±1.0 (n=6031)	131 ± 34 (n=6335)	28.5 ± 4.8 (n=5324)

Table 13. Summary of main findings from large observational study.

EDITORS COMMENTARY

The uncontrolled design of this large study prevents definitive conclusions but nevertheless, the translational message appears clear regarding the clinical value of insulin glargine. These data suggest that, in daily clinical practice, insulin glargine in combination with OHAs is a simple and highly effective strategy to achieve good glycemic control in patients with T2DM inadequately controlled on OHAs alone. This is consistent with the results seen in many clinical trials. The mean HBA$_{1c}$ recorded at 9 months documented that the target of ≤7% was achieved. Considering the magnitude of this study conducted in more than 12000 patients, it is surprising that only 19 adverse events due to hypoglycemia were reported and there was no overall change in body weight despite significant improvements in glycemic control.

TREATMENT SATISFACTION AND COSTS

Improved psychological outcomes after initiation of insulin treatment in patients with type 2 diabetes.

Witthaus E, Stewart J, Bradley C. *Diabetologia* 2000; 43(Suppl 1):A205 Abstract 787.

STUDY DESCRIPTION

This represents the additional analysis conducted on subjects enrolled in a registration trial conducted in Europe (Massi Benedetti et al., 2003) and described on page 99. The satisfaction and psychological well-being associated with insulin treatment, either NPH insulin or insulin glargine given once-daily at bedtime was evaluated in this analysis. Data included in this analysis included both insulin naïve (n=318) and insulin pre-treated patients (n=114).

STUDY DESIGN

The majority of subjects (n=432) from the randomized trial completed the Diabetes Treatment Satisfaction Questionnaire (DTSQ) and the Well-being Questionnaire (W-BQ) at baseline and at weeks 8, 20, 36 and 52. An analysis of covariance was conducted on the changes from baseline scores from the two questionnaires. The main effects were treatment and the pooled site (for each country e.g. France) and the covariate was the baseline score.

OBJECTIVES

To assess patients' satisfaction with treatment and psychological well-being in response to insulin treatment, either NPH insulin or insulin glargine administered once-daily at bedtime.

OUTCOME VARIABLES

* Changes from baseline in the DTSQ and W-BQ scores, including assessments of the different components of each score.

KEY FINDINGS

* The "Treatment Satisfaction" component of the DTSQ significantly improved at all time points, including the endpoint (52 weeks) for each insulin treatment group (NPH insulin, $p<0.01$; insulin glargine, $p<0.01$) and was significantly increased at week 36 in the subjects treated with insulin glargine compared to NPH insulin ($p=0.0329$). The most marked increase in score occurred in subjects previously treated with insulin therapy prior to trial enrollment.
* The "Perceived Frequency of Hyperglycemia" component of the DTSQ was significantly reduced at all time points, including the endpoint (52 weeks) with each insulin treatment category (NPH insulin, $p<0.01$; insulin glargine, $p<0.01$).
* The "Perceived Frequency of Hypoglycemia" component of the DTSQ significantly increased with insulin treatment ($p<0.01$), but there was no difference between the groups.
* W-BQ did not change during the study period and was similar for the two treatment groups.

EDITORS COMMENTARY

The analysis showed greater treatment satisfaction among patients receiving insulin glargine compared to NPH insulin. This improvement in treatment satisfaction among insulin glargine treated patients was higher than with NPH insulin at week 36 (p=0.03) with a trend towards better treatment satisfaction in the insulin glargine group at the study end (p=0.06). Furthermore, within each treatment group, satisfaction increased over time for all time points (p<0.01 vs. baseline). In addition, the insulin pre-treated patients (n=114) who were randomized to insulin glargine showed a greater increase in treatment satisfaction from baseline compared with patients treated with NPH insulin. The perceived frequency of hyperglycemia was reduced at all time points with both treatments. However, there was no change over time in "Well-Being Questionnaire" scores either within, or between, each treatment group.

Abstract

Influence of patient experience with insulin glargine on trade-offs between glycemic control and hypoglycemia: an analysis of the treat-to-target trial.

Johnson FR, Hauber AB, Bolinder B. *Diabetes* 2004; 53(Suppl 2):Abstract 1166-P.

STUDY DESCRIPTION

Willingness to improve glycemic control is intrinsically related to fear of hypoglycemia which is a major insulin barrier. Patients are often willing to trade better glycemic control in an attempt to reduce the risk of hypoglycemia. The extent of this "trade-off" as influenced by previous insulin treatment experience was compared between insulin glargine and NPH. This additional analysis of a subgroup of insulin naive patients with T2DM (n=381) enrolled in the 24-week, randomized controlled "treat-to-target" trial (Riddle, Rosenstock and Gerich, 2003) compared once-daily NPH insulin with insulin glargine. Randomized patients completed a sequence of three versions of a self-administered, choice-format conjoint survey at the beginning, midpoint and end of the study. Estimated ordered probit coefficients of patient preferences were obtained at baseline and endpoint.

OBJECTIVES

To quantify changes in patients' views of the trade-off between better glycemic control and hypoglycemia at the beginning and end of the "treat-to-target" trial.

KEY FINDINGS

- At baseline, all patients expressed a clear preference for improving glucose control and avoiding nocturnal hypoglycemia, which was comparable between the two treatment groups.
- At baseline, patients perceived that lowering the incidence of hypoglycemia by one event/month was equivalent to a 23.5 mg/dL (90% confidence interval [CI] 32.5, 15.6) improvement in FPG in insulin glargine-treated patients, and a 30.8 mg/dL (90% CI 39.5, 20.7) improvement in FPG in NPH-treated patients, which were not significantly different.

- At the study endpoint, patients treated with insulin glargine were more willing to improve their glucose control in response to reductions in the incidence of nocturnal hypoglycemia compared to NPH-treated patients.

- At endpoint, reducing hypoglycemic episodes by one event/month was perceived as equivalent to significantly greater FPG improvements of 29.5 mg/dL (90% CI 38.7, 20.7) in the insulin glargine group compared to 13.3 mg/dL (90% CI 20.7, 6.8) with NPH insulin.

EDITORS COMMENTARY

Patients are often willing to compromise their glucose control to reduce the level of hypoglycemia they experience and this is influenced by treatment experience. This study wished to examine how the perception of patients changed during the course of the "treat-to-target" study during which patients received either insulin glargine or NPH insulin. As expected, at study entry patients expressed a clear preference for avoiding nocturnal hypoglycemia in both treatment groups. The analysis suggested that over the 24-week treatment with insulin glargine, fear of hypoglycemia and patients' willingness to improve glycemic control improved compared to NPH insulin treatment. This is encouraging and also suggests that insulin glargine treatment may lead to better treatment compliance.

Analysis of a managed care population: relationship between paid hypoglycemia claim rate and reported A_{1c} levels in patients initiated on long-acting insulin (Glargine) or intermediate-acting insulin (NPH).

Al-Zakwani I, Bullano MF, Menditto L, Vincent J. Willey VJ. *Diabetes* 2004; 53(Suppl 2): Abstract 2029-PO.

Abstract

STUDY DESCRIPTION

This was a retrospective cohort study conducted in the United States. A 2.5 million-member managed care integrated medical and pharmacy administrative claims and laboratory results database was examined for hypoglycemia claims over a 2.5 year time period.

STUDY DESIGN

Patients newly initiated on insulin (n=1434), either glargine (n=310) or NPH (n=1124) between July 2000 and August 2002 were identified. Hypoglycemia claims were identified via ICD-9 codes. Negative binomial regression model techniques were utilized in an attempt to predict hypoglycemia claims, which is a similar modeling method to Poisson estimation, used previously to compare the risk of hypoglycemia between insulin glargine and NPH insulin (Yki-Jarvinen et al., 2003; Riddle et al., 2004). The hypoglycemia claim rate was generated from the model by varying HbA_{1c} and keeping other covariates constant. The covariates used in the analysis included age, gender, baseline hypoglycemia claims, regular insulin use, oral hypoglycemic agents, and lowest reported HbA_{1c}.

OBJECTIVES

To compare differences in paid hypoglycemia claim rates identified in a medical claims database, with respect to reported HbA_{1c} values within a managed care population newly initiated on insulin with either NPH insulin or insulin glargine.

KEY FINDINGS

- A total of 88 claims relating to hypoglycemia were recorded.

- For patients newly initiated to insulin treatment, NPH insulin was 3 times more likely to be associated with a higher hypoglycemia claim rate than insulin glargine (IRR 3.18, 95% CI: 1.33 to 7.62).

- At a reported HbA_{1c}, patients newly initiated to NPH insulin had a higher paid hypoglycemia claim rate compared to insulin glargine treatment.

EDITORS COMMENTARY

The predicted mean hypoglycemia rate as a function of reported HbA_{1c} was clearly greater with NPH. Furthermore, NPH showed a steeper increment in predicted hypoglycemia, widening the difference with insulin glargine that had a relatively flat curve with no substantial increment of predicted hypoglycemia with HbA_{1c} levels in the 5% to 7% range. This analysis of hypoglycemia claims made to a managed care program showed that the claim rates in patients treated with insulin are reduced in patients receiving insulin glargine compared to NPH insulin. The analysis does not distinguish between T1DM and T2DM. The findings of this negative binomial regression analysis that the hypoglycemia claim rate is higher for a given HbA_{1c} for patients treated with NPH insulin are in keeping with the Poisson regression analyses that have been conducted in subjects enrolled in clinical studies assessing the efficacy and safety of insulin glargine compared to NPH insulin (Yki-Jarvinen et al., 2003; Riddle et al., 2004). This reduction of hypoglycemia claims with insulin glargine provides objective evidence on potential cost savings. However, the major potential savings impact, which is difficult to quantify in health economics, is on the reduction of fear of hypoglycemia.

Abstract

Pharmacoeconomic analysis of insulin glargine compared with NPH insulin in patients with type 2 diabetes in Spain.

Terrés CR, Rodríguez J, Bolinder B, De Pablos P. *Diabetes* 2004; 53(Suppl 2):Abstract 1197-P.

STUDY DESCRIPTION

This was a retrospective, cost-utility analysis (CUA) using a deterministic model based on the Spanish National Health System. The impact of treatment was measured both in monetary terms and the outcome expressed in terms of patient preferences or quality of life. Quality adjustments are based on a series of preference weights that reflect the importance patients place on different states of health. In this model, the analysis was conducted on a hypothetical patient population with baseline characteristics based on results from the UKPDS and with a simulation of the course of T2DM over a 10 year period.

STUDY DESIGN

Event probabilities, resource utilization and direct costs were inferred from the UKPDS, comparative clinical trials, and from a Spanish health cost database. Health utility values, including Quality-Adjusted Life Years (QALYs), the preferred measure used in CUA analyses, were obtained from the Cost of Diabetes in Europe – Type 2 (CODE-2) study. Univariate and multivariate sensitivity analyses were performed.

OBJECTIVES

To compare the cost-effectiveness of insulin glargine and NPH insulin in patients with T2DM in Spain.

KEY FINDINGS

- According to this model, the average additional health utilities with insulin glargine compared to NPH insulin were +0.238 QALYs (with discount applied) and +0.254 QALYs (without discount applied).

- The additional cost per QALY obtained with insulin glargine was €9243 and €10,969, with and without discounts, respectively. These were based on 2002 prices.

- The sensitivity analyses confirmed the robustness of the base case analysis, with costs per QALY of €2000–11,000, except when the impact of the fear of hypoglycemia was excluded. Ignoring the hypoglycemia fear resulted in costs per QALY exceeding €30,000.

EDITORS COMMENTARY

This was an hypothetical exercise but nevertheless, the analysis showed favorable cost-effectiveness was shown for insulin glargine, which was driven by a number of parameters with respect to treatment efficacy, including a lower incidence of severe hypoglycemia and with possible improvements in HbA_{1c} compared to NPH insulin. These costs per QALY gained are well within the acceptable threshold in Spain of €30,000 per QALY gained.

Future economic evaluations, such as CUA, are important to conduct as they provide insight into the overall cost of therapeutic interventions and allow comparisons of the different consequences in terms of quantity and quality of life, expressed as utilities, such as QALYs. In Spain, insulin glargine appears at least theoretically a cost-effective alternative to NPH insulin in patients with T2DM, with more QALYs gained and costs reduced due to fewer complications compared to NPH insulin.

INCOMPLETE STUDIES

Basal insulin therapy in type 2 diabetes: A prospective 18-month comparison of insulin glargine and NPH insulin in patients with a multiple injection regimen.

Siegmund T, Born T, Weber S, Usadel KH, Schumm-Draeger PM. *Diabetes* 2003; 52(Suppl 1): A456 Abstract 1976-PO.

STUDY DESCRIPTION

This is an ongoing long-term single center open-label comparison of the efficacy and safety of once-daily insulin glargine with twice-daily NPH insulin in persons with T2DM receiving short-acting pre-prandial insulin analogs, undertaken over an 18-month period. Findings from an initial 103 patients have been reported.

KEY FINDINGS TO DATE

Baseline to endpoint mean HbA_{1c} was significantly reduced with insulin glargine from 7.4 to 7% (mean reduction ($\pm$ SD): $0.39 \pm 0.8\%$; $p<0.003$) but not with NPH insulin (7.4 to 7.2%: mean reduction $0.2 \pm 0.78\%$; p=NS). There was no significant increase in the daily insulin dose or in the pre-prandial insulin doses (NPH group dose (U/kg): start dose: 0.35, final dose: 0.38; insulin glargine start dose: 0.28, final dose: 0.29). Patient body weight remained unchanged. A higher number of symptomatic hypoglycemic events occurred with NPH insulin compared to insulin glargine. No severe hypoglycemic events were recorded.

EDITORS COMMENTARY

Given that there is little data on the long-term use of insulin glargine in persons with T2DM, especially in those using multiple injection regimens, this study will offer useful data on long-term outcomes in persons receiving intensive insulin therapy. In the preliminary findings presented, insulin glargine-treated patients showed significant improvement in glycemic control over an 18-month period, with a reduction in mean HbA_{1c} to target levels of 7% with no weight gain and no severe hypoglycemic events described in any patient.

Patients with type 2 diabetes do not receive adequate diabetes education despite presence of neuropathy and other diabetic complications.

M. Pfeifer, L. Kennedy, W. Herman for the GOAL A1C Study Group. *Diabetes Metabolism* 2003; 29(Spec No2): Abstract.

STUDY DESCRIPTION

The GOAL A1C (**G**lycemia **O**ptimization with **A**lgorithms and **L**abs **A**t Po**1**nt of **C**are) study is enrolling 14000 insulin-naïve persons with T2DM inadequately controlled on OHAs to insulin glargine, in the primary care setting is to assess point-of-care testing within the context of "treat-to-target" insulin dosing plan.

KEY FINDINGS TO DATE

Preliminary findings on the education received by 3578 patients have been presented.

EDITORS COMMENTARY

The findings of the use of insulin glargine in everyday practice will offer insight into the value of this innovative approach involving primary care physicians, insulin dosing algorithms and near patient testing to lower FBG and achieve glycemic targets.

Abstract

Basal supported oral therapy (BOT) in everyday practice.

Janka HU, Schneider K, Schweitzer MA. *Diabetes Metabolism* 2003; 29(Spec No 2): Abstract 2206.

STUDY DESCRIPTION

This ongoing observational single clinical practice study is enrolling a large group of persons with T2DM inadequately controlled by OHA who are being instigated onto insulin glargine. Decisions regarding treatment and dosing are made at the discretion of physicians, to reflect everyday clinical practice.

KEY FINDINGS TO DATE

In the initial report from this study of 1958 patients, FBG was reduced from 11 ± 3.1 mmol/L at baseline to 7.3 ± 1.7 mmol/L at 3 months. HbA_{1c} was reduced from $8.8 \pm 2.5\%$ at baseline to $7.3 \pm 1.0\%$ at 3 months. Mean body weight remained stable with a tendency towards weight reduction (-0.6 ± 3.0 kg). The mean insulin dose increased from $13.7 \pm$ 7.0 U at baseline to 18.3 ± 8.4 U at 3 months. The physician-assessed compliance has been good or very good in almost 90% of patients. At 3 months, 95% of patients had elected to remain on insulin glargine therapy.

EDITORS COMMENTARY

The preliminary findings from this study suggest that insulin glargine therapy improves metabolic control safely without causing weight gain in persons with T2DM poorly controlled by OHA in the setting of everyday clinical practice. Furthermore, it seems that concerns about the introduction of insulin therapy are being overcome with high levels of treatment satisfaction and compliance recorded.

Improvement of brittle diabetes control after switching to insulin glargine (Lantus®) from NPH insulin: a continuous glucose monitoring study.

Levin P, Soumai M, Lee F, Mersey J. *Diabetes Metabolism* 2003; 29(Spec No2);Abstract 2218.

STUDY DESCRIPTION

This ongoing single center study is being conducted in persons with "brittle" T2DM i.e. persons who experience difficulties in establishing glycemic stability and suffer frequent episodes of hypoglycemia with wide and unstable fluctuations in BG. The study aims to determine the effect of switching basal insulin support from NPH insulin to insulin glargine by measuring the occurrence of hypoglycemia using continuous glucose monitoring, and assessing glycemic stability. In the study, patients undergo continuous glucose monitoring (CGM) for a period of 3 days while receiving their existing basal insulin therapy of twice-daily injections of NPH insulin supplemented by occasional additional mealtime insulin or metformin. Patients then receive insulin glargine, titrated using an established protocol to a fasting blood glucose level of <100 mg/dL (5.5 mmol/L). Following titration of the insulin glargine dose, patients undergo a second 3 day period of CGM.

KEY FINDINGS TO DATE

The preliminary findings from eight patients reported a 15% reduction in average BG and a 34% reduction in total average hypoglycemia time following the switch from NPH insulin to insulin glargine.

Abstract

Feasibility of improved glycemic control with insulin detemir and insulin glargine in combination with oral agents in insulin naive patients with type 2 diabetes.

Rosenstock J, Larsen J, Draeger E, Kristensen HS, Davies M. *Diabetes* 2004; 53(Suppl 2): Abstract 610-P.

Long acting insulin analogs with protracted, predictable and flat profiles are ideal candidates for basal insulin replacement added to OHAs in T2DM to attain and sustain the stringent new guidelines for target with less risk of hypoglycemia. Of interest in this trial is the first carefully designed head to head comparison of the 2 long acting insulin analogs, insulin detemir and insulin glargine to assess effects on glycemic control, weight and hypoglycemia. This open-label, multicenter trial is designed to compare the efficacy and safety of insulin detemir and insulin glargine in the treatment of insulin naïve subjects (n=582) with T2DM who have been treated with OHAs for at least 4 months (excluding thiazolidinediones). Patients continued their current OHA treatment and were randomized to either insulin detemir (given at bedtime, and additionally, if required, in the morning) or insulin glargine, once-daily only at bedtime, for a period of one year. The insulin dose was titrated according to a structured and forced algorithm with a target pre-breakfast PG and pre-dinner PG (PDPG) of ≤108 mg/dL (6 mmol/L) (Table 14), based on 3 self-measured FPG values. The additional morning dose of insulin detemir was allowed if the PDPG remained above 126 mg/dL (7 mmol/L) once the FPG < 126 mg/dL was achieved. This additional insulin detemir dose was adjusted using a specific algorithm that was based on 3 self-measured PDPG values (Table 15). Starting doses of evening basal insulin were the same for both insulins at 12 U.

KEY FINDINGS TO DATE

A total of 582 patients were randomized, but preliminary findings from only 120 patients treated for 28 weeks are presented. The mean FPG improved from 178 ± 45 mg/dL (9.9 ± 2.5 mmol/L) at trial entry to 108 ± 23 mg/dL (6.0 ± 1.3 mmol/L) after 28 weeks (p<0.01), with 63% of patients reaching target FPG ≤108 mg/dL (6 mmol/L). The mean PDPG was lowered from 178 ± 58 mg/dL (9.9 ± 3.2 mmol/L) to 117 ± 39 mg/dL (6.5 ± 2.2 mmol/L) (p<0.01).

Average pre-breakfast PG	Change in insulin dose (U)
>180 mg/dL (>10.0 mmol/L)	12
163–180 mg/dL (9.1–10.0 mmol/L)	8
145–162 mg/dL (8.1–9.0 mmol/L)	6
127–144 mg/dL (7.1–8.0 mmol/L)	4
109–126 mg/dL (6.1–7.0 mmol/L)	2
<108 mg/dL (<6.0 mmol/L)	0

Table 14. Dose algorithm based on FPG.

Average pre-dinner PG	Change in detemir dose (U)
>180 mg/dL (>10.0 mmol/L)	8
163–180 mg/dL (9.1–10.0 mmol/L)	6
145–162 mg/dL (8.1–9.0 mmol/L)	4
127–144 mg/dL (7.1–8.0 mmol/L)	2
109–126 mg/dL (6.1–7.0 mmol/L)	2
<108 mg/dL (<6.0 mmol/L)	0

Table 15. Dose algorithm based on PDPG.

EDITORS COMMENTARY

This important head-to-head study, planned to compare the relative efficacy of the long acting insulin analogs insulin detemir and insulin glargine, awaits full completion. This study involves two basal insulins with different principles for retarding the absorption of insulin from subcutaneous tissue. Insulin detemir is an acylated derivative of human insulin with protracted action due to the fatty acid side chain allowing binding with tissue-bound albumin at the injection site, leading to prolongation of action. In contrast the method of insulin glargine retardation relies on the formation of an amorphous precipitate in the subcutaneous tissue delaying absorption.

These initial findings suggest that most patients can achieve FPG targets with administration of these two long acting insulin analogs by adherence to simple dosing algorithms. Most notably, the study design allows for both insulins to maximize their effects according to their reported durations of action. Insulin glargine will be delivered only once a day in keeping with its estimated 24 hour duration whereas insulin detemir that appears to have a shorter duration of action than insulin glargine will be allowed to have a second morning injection but only according some specific glucose parameters. Of great interest is the assessment of the PDPG levels that could provide valuable information on the estimated effective duration of action of both insulins and what percentage of detemir patients will require a second insulin injection. The current feasibility report with both insulins combined showed significant improvement of the PDPG from178 ± 58 mg/dL to 117 ± 39 mg/dL but full comparative analyses between insulin detemir and insulin glargine are awaited upon full completion of the trial. This study should clarify how effective both insulins are in achieving FPG and HbA$_{1c}$ targets and any differences in weight and frequency of hypoglycemia.

Comparison of twice-daily biphasic insulin aspart 70/30 (BIAsp 70/30) with once-daily insulin glargine (GLA) in patients with type 2 DM on oral antidiabetic agents.

Raskin P, Rojas P, Allen E. *Diabetes* 2004; 53(Suppl 2):Abstract 602-P.

Abstract

STUDY DESCRIPTION

This ongoing randomized, open-label, 28-week study has enrolled 233 insulin-naïve patients poorly controlled (HbA$_{1C}$ ≥8.0%) on their current treatment of metformin (≥1000 mg/day), alone or in combination with other OHAs. The metformin dose was adjusted to ≥1500 mg/day during a 4-week run-in period. The patients were then randomized to one of two insulin treatments, either 70/30 insulin twice-daily (morning and suppertime) initiated at 6 U or insulin glargine at bedtime initiated at 10 U. The insulin dose was titrated to a target BG range of 80 - 110 mg/dl (4.4 – 6.1 mmol/L) by a structured and forced algorithm. Dose adjustment was carried out weekly for the first 12 weeks and every 2 weeks thereafter. The suppertime 70/30 insulin dose and the bedtime insulin glargine dose were titrated on the basis of the mean FBG over the previous 3 days. The morning 70/30 insulin dose was titrated on the basis of the mean pre-dinner BG over the previous 3 days.

KEY FINDINGS TO DATE

Findings from 171 patients are reported. At baseline, patient characteristics, including prior OHA treatment, demographics, and HbA$_{1C}$ values were similar between treatment groups. Provisional 28-week findings show that the mean HbA$_{1C}$ was lower in the 70/30 insulin treatment group compared to the insulin glargine group (6.8 ± 0.9% vs. 7.2 ± 0.9, respectively). More 70/30 insulin-treated patients compared to insulin glargine reached the target HbA$_{1C}$ of ≤6.5% (46 vs. 30%, respectively) and HbA$_{1C}$ of <7.0% (71 vs. 45%, respectively). No major hypoglycemic episodes were reported for either treatment group. There was a greater weight gain associated with 70/30 insulin (22.9 ± 25.1 kg vs. 12.5 ± 22.2 kg, respectively).

EDITORS COMMENTARY

This randomized study, undertaken in insulin naïve patients, shows improved glycemic control with 70/30 insulin premix compared to insulin glargine, with a greater number reaching glycemic targets. However, no detailed information is provided regarding the hypoglycemic profile experienced by the patients, and we do not know the insulin doses used. It seems likely that the insulin glargine-treated subjects did not experience effective dose escalation, as shown by the HbA$_{1C}$ levels described. Only after effective titration of the insulin glargine dose can the relative rate of hypoglycemia be accurately ascertained and the impact of these results fully interpreted. It is noteworthy that both treatment groups experienced weight gain, and this was markedly higher in those subjects treated with premixed insulin compared to insulin glargine.

SUMMARY

A more integrated understanding of the pathophysiologic course of T2DM and the clear awareness of the long-term consequences of hyperglycemia has emphasized the need for effective treatment strategies. Insulin therapy is increasingly seen as a key intervention in T2DM in an attempt to reach glycemic targets to prevent the onset and progression of vascular complications related to T2DM.

We have summarized a relatively large clinical trial program that has investigated insulin glargine as basal insulin therapy in persons with T2DM. In these studies, insulin glargine was administered subcutaneously once-daily at bedtime or in the morning, alone and/or in conjunction with OHA and/or short-acting insulin preparations. The program of phase I, II, III, IV and V trials has explored various efficacy, safety and quality-of-life findings. Efficacy parameters have largely been based on FPG, FBG, and HbA_{1c} as indices of glycemic control and on the frequency of hypoglycemia, especially of nocturnal hypoglycemia.

FINDINGS FROM PHASE II STUDIES

Two early phase II studies of short duration (Raskin et al., 1998; page 98; HOE901/2004 Study Investigators Group, 2003; page 95) were initiated to establish the short-term efficacy and safety of insulin glargine (two different formulations) compared to NPH insulin.

In these studies, patients poorly controlled by their existing therapy with OHA were randomized to treatment with NPH insulin or one of two formulations of insulin glargine, which differed in their zinc content (containing either 30 or 80 µg/ml). One such study was conducted in the USA (Raskin et al., 1998) and the other in Europe and South America (HOE901/2004 Study Investigators Group, 2003). Insulin glargine was as effective as NPH insulin in reducing FBG (the primary efficacy

variable), was well tolerated and, in the European study, significantly reduced the frequency of nocturnal hypoglycemia compared to NPH insulin. No clinically relevant differences were observed between the two formulations of insulin glargine. Ultimately, the 30µg/ml zinc formulation was selected for use in the subsequent trial program and as the final product formulation. The importance of zinc in insulin hexamerization was described in Chapter Two (see page 29).

FINDINGS FROM PRINCIPAL PHASE III/IIIB STUDIES

Four randomized, controlled clinical studies have provided the core evidence on the efficacy and safety of insulin glargine providing basal insulin supplementation in persons with T2DM. Two early trials (phase III) were conducted primarily as registration studies. Patients enrolled had been pre-treated with OHAs, alone or in conjunction with insulin (Massi Benedetti et al., 2003) or with insulin alone (Rosenstock et al., 2001). Two further post-registration (phase IIIB) studies were subsequently conducted in insulin naïve subjects with T2DM that examined the potential benefit of adding insulin to oral hypoglycemic agents targeting a lower FBG (100 mg/dL, 5.5 mmol/L) in an attempt to achieve the HbA_{1c} target of 7%. All studies were of a parallel group design and were carried out in a non-blind manner.

Phase III studies

Two principal randomized phase III clinical trials, conducted for registration purposes for the approval of insulin glargine as therapy in persons with T2DM, demonstrate the impact of insulin glargine in insulin naïve patients and also patients previously treated with insulin, predominantly NPH insulin.

The largest study of 52 weeks duration described findings in both insulin-naïve (Yki-Järvinen et al., 2000; page 102) and insulin pre-treated subjects (complete study findings are described by Massi Benedetti et al., 2003; page 99), who had been treated with OHAs. Further sub-analyses were also conducted, which included a comparison of insulin glargine with NPH insulin in obese patients (BMI>28 kg/m²)(Massi Benedetti et al., 2003). An extended non-randomized phase of the study assessed the efficacy and safety of insulin glargine therapy for up to 40 months treatment duration (Kacerovsky-Bielesz and Hirtz, 2002; page 104).

This study showed a significant improvement in glycemic control from baseline to endpoint in subjects receiving insulin glargine and a similar improvement with NPH insulin. Importantly, insulin glargine was associated with a significantly reduced frequency of confirmed nocturnal hypoglycemia. These findings were consistent, regardless of whether subjects had received prior insulin therapy. Other findings included a significantly greater improvement in glycemic control with insulin glargine in the obese subgroup of subjects and a sustained improvement in glycemic control with a low incidence of adverse events in the extended phase of the study.

An important observation in this study was a general inability to achieve the stated FBG target of 120 mg/dL (6.7 mmol/L), which reflects subjects failing to receive adequate insulin supplementation. The study protocol specified that insulin doses were at the discretion of investigators and did not include a formal or structured titration algorithm. As a result, investigators may have failed to sufficiently increase the insulin dose to achieve the target FBG, possibly due to a fear of inducing hypoglycemia.

The second phase III registration trial (Rosenstock et al., 2001; page 106) further explored the comparative efficacy and safety of insulin glargine with NPH insulin. This study was conducted in a group of persons with T2DM who had previously received insulin therapy for more than three months with no concomitant OHAs. Patients received either insulin glargine once-daily at bedtime or NPH insulin, administered once or twice daily, with or without pre-prandial insulin for 28 weeks. Both treatments were associated with similar, significant improvements in glycemic control. However, the incidence of confirmed nocturnal hypoglycemia was significantly lower (25%) in patients treated with insulin glargine. As in the previous study, HbA_{1c} was not reduced to levels below 7.0%, despite titration of the insulin dose up to a median total daily insulin dose of 0.75 U/kg. This may relate to the reluctance of investigators to increase insulin dose due to fears of hypoglycemia or weight gain.

Phase IIIB studies

The seminal study entitled "treat-to-target" explored how insulin glargine might be more effectively deployed in the management of T2DM by testing if lower FBG targets and, potentially, better glycemic control could be achieved through a more aggressive dosing regimen (Riddle, Rosenstock and Gerich, 2003; page 115). This key study enrolled 756 overweight patients (mean BMI>30 kg/m²) poorly controlled by OHAs to receive, in addition to OHAs, either NPH insulin or insulin glargine at bedtime for 24 weeks. The study was designed to show the validity of the "treat-to-target" concept, namely that forced titration of the insulin dose to a FPG target of ≤100mg/dL (5.5 mmol/L) using a simple dosing algorithm allows target glycemic control to be achieved (HbA_{1c} ≤7.0%) in most patients without an accompanying increase in the frequency of hypoglycemia.

The results of the study demonstrated that about 60% of patients in both treatment groups (insulin glargine or NPH insulin) achieved the target HbA_{1c} level of ≤7.0%, but that a significantly greater proportion (25%) of subjects in the insulin glargine group did so without any occurrence of a single confirmed episode of nocturnal hypoglycemia. This study reports that starting insulin therapy with a low dose of 10 U at bedtime, followed by a simple dosing algorithm based on FPG, was successful in achieving impressive improvements in glycemic control. The mean insulin doses at study endpoint were

47 and 42 units per day. The findings confirm the "treat-to-target" concept and underline the potential for translating the insulin dose adjustment regimen into everyday clinical practice, given the simplicity of the treatment and its monitoring (only one FBG measurement required for the purpose of insulin dose adjustment) and the lower frequency of hypoglycemia perceived as the main barrier to insulin dose adjustment, relative to NPH insulin.

Another phase IV study utilized an insulin titration in an attempt to achieve a lower FBG target of 100 mg/dL (5.5 mmol/L) in the context of a simple treatment regimen. This involved a single daily dose of the sulfonylurea, glimepiride, and a single daily injection of insulin, either NPH insulin at bedtime or insulin glargine either in the morning or at bedtime (Fritsche et al., 2003; page 111). Significant improvements in glycemic control occurred in all three treatment groups (bedtime NPH insulin, bedtime insulin glargine and morning insulin glargine). The findings are very interesting because they show that patients receiving morning insulin glargine achieved a significantly greater mean reduction in HbA_{1c} levels at the end of the 24 week study period. Morning insulin glargine was associated with a significantly greater improvement compared to NPH insulin at bedtime (-1.24% vs. -0.84%) and also insulin glargine given at bedtime (-0.96%). There was a significantly higher frequency of nocturnal hypoglycemia with NPH insulin (38%) compared to insulin glargine, given either in the morning (17%; p<0.001) or at bedtime (23%; p<0.001).

Taken with the "treat-to-target" study (Riddle, Rosenstock and Gerich, 2003), this latter study suggests that titration of the insulin dose to achieve target FBG levels will result in effective restoration of glycemic control, without incurring an unacceptable level of nocturnal hypoglycemia. Importantly, this can be achieved using a simple combination regimen of "one pill" (e.g. glimepiride) and "one shot" (insulin glargine).

FINDINGS FROM META-ANALYSES OF RANDOMIZED CONTROLLED STUDIES

The principal phase III/IIIB studies offered important data on glycemic control and hypoglycemia with insulin treatment in poorly controlled subjects with T2DM. In an attempt to extend these findings, meta-regression analyses and meta-analyses were conducted on these studies with the goal of further defining the relationship between glycemic control and hypoglycemic side effects.

A meta-regression analysis (Yki-Järvinen et al., 2003; page 119) of three of the principal studies (Massi Benedetti et al., 2003; Riddle, Rosenstock and Gerich, 2003 and Fritsche et al., 2003) confirmed their original findings of achieving glycemic control with reduced hypoglycemia with insulin glargine compared to NPH insulin. The analysis models the effects of insulin glargine and NPH insulin on HbA_{1c} levels when the incidences of hypoglycemia were made equivalent. The larger numbers in the analysis (1785 persons with T2DM) offer greater power than the individual studies alone. This innovative analysis used Poisson regression analysis and predicts that HbA_{1c} levels are 0.44% lower with insulin glargine treatment at a given rate of symptomatic hypoglycemia, compared to once-daily NPH insulin. Most importantly, the model shows that, for a given similar frequency of nocturnal hypoglycemia, the mean HbA_{1c} levels are predicted to be 0.87% lower with insulin glargine, which is clinically significant. These findings are backed by the most recent Poisson analysis of the "treat-to-target" trial, which confirmed the expectation of significantly lower HbA_{1c} with insulin glargine for equivalent levels of nocturnal hypoglycemia (Riddle et al., 2004; page 121).

Two further individual meta-analyses have been reported (Rosenstock et al., 2003; page 123 and Dailey et al., 2003; page 123), which differed with respect to the patients included and the type of analysis conducted. The meta-analyses included 2304 patients from the four principal phase III/IIIB studies (Massi Benedetti et al., 2003; Rosenstock et al., 2001; Riddle, Rosenstock and Gerich, 2003 and Fritsche et al., 2003). The incidence of all symptomatic hypoglycemic and symptomatic nocturnal hypoglycemic episodes, both confirmed and unconfirmed, was significantly lower (all p values <0.001) in the insulin glargine group compared to the NPH insulin group. Considering nocturnal hypoglycemia specifically, patients treated with insulin glargine had a 29% risk reduction compared to NPH insulin. Severe hypoglycemia (PG≤56 mg/dL (3.1 mmol/L)) has been shown to be numerically lower in most insulin glargine studies, but due to the low overall number of episodes was not shown to be significantly different to NPH insulin. However, the meta-analysis from the pooled data demonstrated that episodes of severe hypoglycemia, both overall and nocturnal, are significantly reduced by 19% and 29% respectively with insulin glargine compared to NPH insulin.

Taken together, the four analyses reveal significant and clinically relevant improvements in glycemic control associated with insulin glargine therapy. The analyses performed separately by Rosenstock and Dailey confirm that insulin glargine is associated with a reduced risk of hypoglycemia and imply that lower FBG targets and hence improved glycemic control are potentially possible using insulin glargine.

The clinical trials and these additional analyses provide a substantial body of evidence that indicates benefits with the introduction of insulin treatment in persons with T2DM failing on diet and OHAs and, in particular, with insulin glargine compared to NPH insulin.

FINDINGS FROM QUALITY OF LIFE ANALYSES

The additional benefits of insulin treatment have been formally analyzed in quality of life assessments. An analysis of the registration trial by Massi Benedetti et al., 2003 reported a quality of life assessment. This study was based on a "Diabetes Treatment Satisfaction Questionnaire", which compared treatment satisfaction between insulin glargine and NPH insulin (Witthaus et al., 2000; page 168). Data was collected at weeks 0, 8, 20, 36 and 52 of the study. The results showed greater treatment satisfaction among patients receiving insulin glargine compared to NPH insulin. This improvement in treatment satisfaction among insulin glargine treated patients was significantly greater than with NPH insulin at week 36 (p=0.03) with a trend towards better treatment satisfaction in the insulin glargine group at the study end (p=0.06). Furthermore, within each treatment group, satisfaction increased over time for all time points (p<0.01 vs. baseline). In addition, the insulin-pretreated patients (n=114) who were randomized to insulin glargine showed a greater increase in treatment satisfaction from baseline compared with patients treated with NPH insulin. There was no change over time in "Well-Being Questionnaire" scores within, or between, each treatment group. A supplementary analysis attempted to address how patients' views of the trade-off between better glycemic control and hypoglycemia changed during the "treat-to-target" trial (Johnson et al., 2004; page 170). At entry, the expected finding that patients clearly preferred to avoid nocturnal hypoglycemia was recorded in both treatment groups. Patients in both treatment groups significantly reduced their fear of hyperglycemia more so than hypoglycemia. The analysis suggested that over the 24-week treatment period, insulin glargine-treated patients' willingness to improve glycemic control improved compared to NPH insulin treatment.

It is important to note the devastating effect that an episode of hypoglycemia can have on the quality of life of a person with diabetes and therefore both patients and physicians tend to strive to avoid further episodes. However, this can result in an inevitable compromise or 'trade-off' between a therapeutic strategy employing the adequate dose of insulin to achieve glycemic control and that utilising a dose least likely to cause hypoglycemia. Therefore, hypoglycemia is one of the most significant barriers to achieving the optimal glycemic control needed to reduce the risk of long-term complications of diabetes. As we have described, meta-regression analysis of the principle clinical trials predicts that, for equivalent rates of nocturnal hypoglycemia, insulin glargine is associated with significantly improved glycemic control (HbA_{1c} reduced by 0.87% vs. NPH insulin). This suggests that the use of insulin glargine has the capacity to impact positively on the relationship between hypoglycemia and glycemic control at an individual level. Therefore, the potential exists to substantially improve the overall glycemic burden for those treated with insulin, which has far reaching consequences in terms of long-term health outcomes. This is borne out in our own clinical practice; in many cases, after effective insulin glargine dose escalation using the "treat-to-target" algorithm, the sustained improvement in glycemic control has been associated with reduced fear of hypoglycemia and improved well-being in individual patients.

FINDINGS FROM ADDITIONAL RANDOMIZED TRIALS

A phase IV randomized study confirmed that combining a sulfonylurea with morning or bedtime insulin glargine is an effective strategy for the management of T2DM (Standl et al., 2003; page 125). Equivalent improvements in glycemic control and similar frequencies of nocturnal, symptomatic and severe hypoglycemia occurred with insulin glargine administered in the morning or at bedtime. Additional analysis of the randomized study demonstrated that around half the patients treated with insulin glargine reached the target HbA_{1c} of ≤7% (Standl et al., 2004; page 127) and that there was no difference in the frequency of nocturnal hypoglycemia in those that did or did not reach target. A sub- analysis showed that patients who began the study on a lower dose of glimepiride, implying an earlier stage of T2DM, required less insulin and experienced fewer episodes of hypoglycemia and less weight gain compared to those on higher glimepiride doses, supporting

the benefits of the early introduction of insulin (Fach et al., 2004; page 129). The results of this study, reviewed in conjunction with the study by Fritsche et al., indicate that flexible timing of dosing (AM or PM) with insulin glargine is possible and suggest an advantage in terms of patient compliance. Indeed, insulin glargine is now approved in Europe and the United States for once-daily treatment at anytime of the day.

Two studies have been conducted that extend the findings on the safety and efficacy of insulin glargine from existing clinical trials conducted in European and North American populations to Latin American countries (Eliaschewitz et al., 2003; page 131) and Asia (Pan et al., 2004; page 133).

The Latin American experience confirms those of European and North American studies in that a single daily dose of glimepiride combined with a single daily dose of insulin glargine, actively titrated using the "treat-to-target" algorithm can effectively restore glycemic control in persons with T2DM. In this study, a quarter of patients treated with insulin glargine reached target HbA_{1c} of 7% without a single occurrence of symptomatic confirmed nocturnal hypoglycemia. Overall, the incidence of confirmed nocturnal hypoglycemia was almost halved in the patients who received insulin glargine compared to NPH insulin (30.0% vs.16.9%; p<0.001). The Asian study employed a higher target FBG of 120 mg/dL (6.7 mmol/L) for the dosing algorithm and a smaller reduction in HbA_{1c} in both treatment groups was seen but did confirm the finding of a much lower frequency of hypoglycemia with insulin glargine compared to NPH insulin (620 vs. 221 events; p<0.001).

A number of initial reports have described the efficacy and safety of insulin glargine in comparison to premixed insulin preparations. The SWITCH-PILOT study (Schiel et al., 2003; page 139) was, as the name suggests, a pilot study to investigate the feasibility of switching persons with T2DM receiving conventional insulin therapy consisting of premixed insulins twice-daily to a simpler, more flexible treatment of morning insulin glargine combined with OHA (glimepiride or

Authors	Duration (Weeks)	Patients	Insulin Treatment Groups	Endpoint HbA$_{1c}$ (%)*		P value
				Glargine	**NPH**	
Massi-Benedetti et al., 2003	52	Insulin-naïve; insulin pre-treated	Glargine/ NPH	8.54	8.52	NS
Yki-Järvinen et al., 2000	52	Insulin-naive	Glargine/ NPH	8.3±0.1	8.2±0.1	NS
Kacerovsky-Bielesz and Hirtz, 2002	160	Insulin-naïve; insulin pre-treated	Glargine	8.42	-	-
Rosenstock et al., 2001	28	Insulin pre-treated	Glargine/ NPH	8.19±0.1	7.91±0.1	NS
Fritsche et al., 2003	24	Insulin-naive	Glargine/ NPH	7.8±1.2 (morning) 8.1±1.3 (bedtime)	8.3±1.3	<0.001[a] 0.008[b]
Riddle, Rosenstock and Gerich, 2003	24	Insulin-naive	Glargine/ NPH	6.96	6.97	NS
Standl et al., 2003	28	Insulin-naive	Glargine: Morning/ Bedtime	7.18 morning 7.23 bedtime	–	NS
Eliaschewitz et al., 2003	24	Insulin-naive	Glargine/ NPH	7.7	7.6	NS
Schiel et al., 2003	16	Insulin pre-treated (CIT)	Glargine/ CIT	7.9[c] 7.4[d] 7.8[e]		NS

NS: Not Significant
* Mean ± SEM
[a] morning glargine vs. NPH
[b] morning vs. bedtime glargine
[c] morning glargine plus glimepiride
[d] glargine plus glimepiride plus metformin
[e] CIT

Table 16. Summary of HbA$_{1c}$ levels described in the principal phase III/IIIB studies.

glimepiride plus metformin)). This pilot study showed that the treatments were equally effective at restoring glycemic control and that insulin therapy gained high patient acceptance, with 88% of patients choosing to remain on insulin glargine treatment at the end of the trial.

Further randomized studies have recently extended the data available and begin to offer insight into the relative merits of each of these insulin strategies, namely the use of premixed insulin alone or basal insulin supplementation with OHAs. The "LAPTOP" study (see page 141) compared conventional insulin therapy (CIT) consisting of twice daily premixed insulin (30% regular soluble human insulin, 70% NPH insulin – PreMix) to insulin glargine given once-daily, with continued sulfonylurea and metformin in insulin-naïve patients poorly controlled by OHA (Janka et al., 2004; page 141). The study showed that almost 50% more patients treated with insulin glargine achieved target HbA$_{1c}$ without even a single recorded incidence of hypoglycemia. Less than half the dose of insulin glargine was required to achieve the target FBG of 100 mg/dL (5.5 mmol/L) when compared to the premixed insulin regimen. Importantly, the insulin glargine treatment was more acceptable to patients, resulting in less weight gain and a better adherence to the structured titration required to achieve the FBG target.

Authors	Duration (Weeks)	Patients	Insulin Treatment Groups	Nocturnal Hypoglycemia (%)		P value
				Glargine	NPH	
Massi-Benedetti et al., 2003	52	Insulin-naïve; insulin pre-treated	Glargine/ NPH	12	24	0.0002
Yki-Järvinen et al., 2000	52	Insulin-naive	Glargine/ NPH	9.9	24.0	0.011
Rosenstock et al., 2001	28	Insulin pre-treated	Glargine/ NPH	26.5	35.5	0.0136
Fritsche et al., 2003	24	Insulin-naive	Glargine: Morning/ Bedtime	17 23	38	<0.001 <0.001
Riddle, Rosenstock, and Gerich, 2003	24	Insulin-naive	Glargine/ NPH	4.0	6.9	<0.001
Standl et al., 2003	28	Insulin-naive	Glargine: Morning/ Bedtime	13.0 14.9	–	NS
Eliaschewitz et al., 2003	24	Insulin-naive	Glargine/ NPH	16.9	30.0	<0.001

NS: Not significant

Table 17. Summary of frequency of nocturnal hypoglycemia.

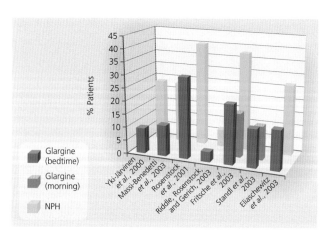

Figure 126. Summary of frequency of nocturnal hypoglycemia.

Three other studies have also attempted to compare insulin glargine to premixed insulin (Malone et al., 2004a; Malone et al., 2004b; Jacober et al., 2004; pages 143, 145, 147). Two studies have compared insulin glargine once-daily at bedtime to twice-daily Humalog Mix 75/25 (75% NPL/25% insulin lispro), both insulins in conjunction with metformin, for a treatment period of 16 weeks, in insulin naïve (Malone et al., 2004a) and insulin exposed (Malone et al., 2004b) patients. The findings from these studies, which have been published as abstracts only, suggest that subjects treated with insulin glargine were not effectively insulinized and did not experience adequate dose escalation. This is borne out by the relatively high glycated hemoglobin and blood glucose values described. Nonetheless, these comparisons are valid and show the ability of insulin therapy to effectively restore glycemic control in persons with T2DM and begin to offer important insights into alternative insulin strategies that are available for patients.

Further studies that aim to extend the findings of the seminal "treat-to-target" study by investigating different, patient-managed algorithms to achieve target blood glucose values have been reported as abstracts and offer insight into how to optimize the initiation and dose titration of insulin (Davies et al., 2004; page149; Lavalle-González et al., 2004; page 151; Yki-Järvinen et al., 2004; page 153). These are discussed in more detail in Chapter 4. These studies are important because, in patients with T2DM who are poorly controlled on oral agents, the insulin dose that is required to restore effective glycemic control is not predictable and is dependent on individual patient characteristics that are not fully defined, but which certainly include the key factor of insulin resistance.

The AT.LANTUS study (see page 149) compared the insulin glargine dose-escalation algorithm previously employed in the "treat-to-target" study with a simpler, patient-led algorithm that required patient self-titration of the insulin glargine dose. This was increased by 2 units every 3 days if FBG was >100 mg/dL (>5.5 mmol/L) and until FBG target was achieved and modulated by the occurrence of severe hypoglycemia. The initial findings from AT.LANTUS suggest that the simpler patient-self managed algorithm achieved better glycemic control with very little difference between the algorithms with respect to frequency of hypoglycemia. Further analyses of this important trial are expected in the near future.

The provisional findings of the recently reported LANMET study (see page 153) are complimentary to the AT.LANTUS and "treat-to-target" studies. LANMET used an almost identical algorithm to the self-titration dose escalation employed in the AT.LANTUS study, but with a lower FPG target of 72 – 100 mg/dL and, as an additional feature, the study required a transfer of FPG values by modem to the treatment center for continuous assessment. The LANMET study compared insulin glargine and NPH insulin in insulin naïve patients poorly controlled on OHA alone, with both treatment groups using this dose escalation algorithm. The findings showed that the mean HbA_{1c} was markedly reduced, almost to target levels (mean 7.1%), but, as expected with a 44% higher incidence of symptomatic hypoglycemia with NPH insulin. The mean insulin doses used to reach this level of glycemic control (68 units of insulin glargine and 70 units of NPH insulin) are markedly higher than the "treat-to-target" study and suggest that this method of patient empowered dose adjustment using an easier algorithm with distant monitoring may be an effective method.

FINDINGS FROM UNCONTROLLED OBSERVATION STUDIES

The findings from randomized clinical trials have been complimented by a series of uncontrolled, observational studies, which aim to determine if the benefits seen in the controlled environment of clinical trials are translated when insulin glargine is used in the "real world" scenario of everyday clinical practice. The studies, both long-term and short-term, have investigated persons with

T2DM who were poorly controlled by their existing therapies (OHA or insulin).

Most of the studies are relatively small (~100 patients) but three short-term studies, two of which have been reported in detail (Klinge et al., 2003; page 161 and Schreiber et al., 2004; page 166) and one which is ongoing (Janka et al., 2003; page 174) have enrolled large numbers of patients (more than 28,000 patients in total). In these large studies, patients initiated onto insulin glargine therapy (single dose, usually at bedtime) were assessed for periods of up to 18 months. Collectively, these observational studies show improved glycemic control with little or no weight gain and a low incidence of hypoglycemia. Significantly, high levels of treatment satisfaction, patient compliance and improved QoL scores were recorded. These studies reflect a growing experience with insulin glargine in clinical practice and appear to demonstrate that the findings seen in clinical trials are translatable to everyday clinical practice.

OTHER KEY NOTE FINDINGS

Bodyweight
Bodyweight changes described in trials are variable. In the registration study of 518 patients (Rosenstock et al., 2001; page 106) there was significantly less weight gain among patients receiving insulin glargine compared to NPH insulin (mean 0.4 vs. 1.4 kg; p<0.0007) at 24 weeks. This will have been due to the reduction in hypoglycemic events experienced by the insulin glargine subjects, thereby limiting the need for additional carbohydrate intake. One year data from the other registration study (Yki-Jarvinen et al., 2000; page 102) showed that insulin naive patients experienced greater mean body weight gain (around 2 kg with both insulins) compared to insulin pre-treated subjects (0.16 – 0.63 kg). Long-term data from this study (Kacerovsky-Bielesz and Hirtz, 2002; page 104) in 239 patients treated with insulin

glargine and OHA showed the gain in mean body weight of about 2 kg remained stable over the 39 months. This gain accompanied an absolute fall in the mean HbA_{1c} level of about 1%. The mean weight gain experienced in patients receiving morning (3.9 kg) or bedtime (3.7 kg) insulin glargine compared to NPH insulin (2.9 kg) (Fritsche et al., 2003; page 111) and in the comparison study of morning or bedtime insulin glargine (Standl et al., 2004; page 129) were similar. In the latter study, patients taking lower glimepiride doses experienced less weight gain at endpoint (2mg: 0.5kg; 3mg: 1.1kg; 4mg: 2.9kg; p=0.0001). The LANMET study (see page 153), which used a lower plasma glucose range of 72 -100 mg/dL and employed high doses of insulin, also described similar mean weight gain with both insulins, insulin glargine (2.6 kg) or NPH insulin (3.5 kg). These findings compare to a 2 kg weight gain in subjects treated with insulin alone and a 2.8 kg gain in subjects treated with insulin and OHA for up to six years in the UKPDS 57 study (Wright et al., 2002). These are summarized in Table 18 and Figure 127.

In the uncontrolled observational studies, improvements in mean HbA_{1c} levels were not accompanied by any statistically significant bodyweight changes. However, of note in these "real-world" studies is the tendancy for no weight increase with insulin glargine. The analysis by Stryjek-Kaminska et al., 2002 (see page 165), which involved 42 obese patients with a mean baseline BMI of 33.2 kg/m^2, showed a minimal increase in mean bodyweight (0.2 kg) over 12 weeks, despite statistically and clinically significant improvements in HbA_{1c} and FBG levels after starting insulin glargine therapy. Of most significance are the findings from the largest observational study conducted by Schreiber and colleagues (2004; page 166), which showed that in more than 12,000 insulin naïve patients poorly controlled on their OHA treatment, mean BMI fell slightly over the 9-month treatment period to 28.5 kg/m^2 with insulin glargine treatment.

Authors	Duration (Weeks)	Patients	Insulin Treatment Groups	Average Body Weight Change (kg)		P value
				NPH	Glargine	
Massi-Benedetti et al., 2003	52	Insulin-naïve; insulin pre-treated	Glargine/ NPH	+2.34	+2.57	NS
Yki-Järvinen et al., 2000	52	Insulin-naive	Glargine/ NPH	+1.98	+2.01	NS
Kacerovsky-Bielesz and Hirtz, 2002	160	Insulin-naïve; insulin pre-treated	Glargine	–	+2.02	–
Rosenstock et al., 2001	28	Insulin pre-treated	Glargine/ NPH	+1.4	+0.4	<0.0007
Fritsche et al., 2003	24	Insulin-naive	Glargine/ NPH	+2.9	+3.9 (morning) +3.7 (bedtime)	NS
Riddle, Rosenstock, and Gerich, 2003	24	Insulin-naive	Glargine/ NPH	+2.8	+3.0	NS

NS: Not significant

Table 18. Summary of body weight changes in principal phase III/IIIB studies.

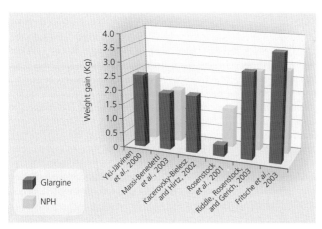

Glargine
NPH

Figure 127. Summary of body weight changes in principal phase III/IIIB studies.

Authors	Duration (Weeks)	Patients	Insulin Treatment Groups	Findings on antibodies to insulins or *E.coli*
Massi-Benedetti et al., 2003	52	Insulin-naïve; insulin pre-treated	Glargine/NPH	The change in levels of antibodies to insulin glargine and human insulin (NPH) was significantly less in insulin glargine-treated patients (p=0.0001). Antibodies to *E. coli* were detected in just a few patients in each treatment group.
Yki-Järvinen et al., 2000	52	Insulin-naive	Glargine/NPH	Antibodies to insulin glargine and human insulin (NPH) were significantly less prevalent in insulin glargine-treated patients
Kacerovsky-Bielesz and Hirtz, 2002	160	Insulin-naïve; insulin pre-treated	Glargine	Antibodies to insulin glargine increased from a mean level of 9.58% (B/T)* at baseline to 11.18% (B/T) at 12 months but decreased to 10.4% (B/T) at the endpoint of the extended study. No trend was observed between *E. coli* antibody titers and adverse events.
Rosenstock et al., 2001	28	Insulin pre-treated	Glargine/NPH	A significantly greater decrease in insulin antibody levels occurred in insulin glargine-treated patients.

B/T: Bound/Total

Table 19. Summary of antibody levels in the principal phase III studies.

Tolerability

In general, apart from the significant differences in the frequency of hypoglycemic episodes, the incidence of adverse events reported in those receiving insulin glargine was similar to subjects treated with NPH insulin. Injection site reactions are the most common adverse events and are seen in 3 - 4% of patients. Long term findings from the extension of The 3002 Study Group (Kacerovsky-Bielesz and Hirtz, 2002) described no injection site reactions over 39 months treatment with insulin glargine. There is no recorded incidence of injection site discomfort with insulin glargine or NPH insulin having resulted in subject withdrawal.

Antibody production

The use of insulin analogs produced using recombinant DNA technology is potentially associated with the development of insulin-binding antibodies and antibodies to *E. coli*. No evidence has been obtained showing clinically relevant changes in levels of either insulin-binding antibodies or antibodies to *E. coli* in patients receiving insulin glargine compared to NPH insulin. In the registration trial of one year duration, the increases seen in insulin-binding antibody production was higher with NPH insulin compared to insulin glargine (p<0.001)(Massi Benedetti et al., 2003).

Patient subgroups – renal impairment

The effect of renal impairment on the pharmacokinetics of insulin glargine has not been studied. Recent data from patients undergoing dialysis for end-stage renal disease who were being treated with insulin glargine revealed no tolerability concerns (Pscherer et al., 2002). It is well recognized that renal impairment reduces the clearance of insulin, necessitating a reduction of the dose in order to reduce hypoglycemia.

EDITORS CONCLUSION

The efficacy and safety of insulin glargine as basal insulin therapy in persons with T2DM is supported by a relatively large body of clinical evidence which demonstrates effective metabolic control and reduced risk of hypoglycemia, relative to NPH insulin. Improved glycemic control is therefore achievable through a simple and flexible "treat-to-target" dose titration regimen, which is translatable to clinical practice.

USING EARLY BASAL INSULIN SUPPLEMENTATION – THE "TREAT-TO-TARGET" PARADIGM

INTRODUCING INSULIN IN T2DM

"Intravenous injections of extract from dog's pancreas, removed from seven to ten weeks after ligation of the ducts, invariably exercises a reducing influence upon the percentage sugar of the blood and the amount of sugar excreted in the urine.... The extent and duration of the reduction varies directly with the amount of extract injected."

Banting FG, Best CH. *J Lab Clin Med* 1922; 7:251–266.

Much has evolved since this epoch-making discovery in the understanding of DM and the seminal role of insulin as the most powerful therapeutic agent transforming management and outcome, limited only by hypoglycemia. Despite this, it is now widely acknowledged that healthcare providers are sub-optimally utilizing insulin in the care of people with DM, thereby withholding the full potential benefit and therefore failing to limit and or eradicate the distressing and disabling complications related to DM. This scenario is certainly the situation confronting the majority of persons with T2DM, who need insulin to normalize their grossly dysmetabolic milieu and poor quality of life, uncorrectable by diet and a variety of OHAs in different combinations. Although this is increasingly recognized, the intervention strategies remain invariably too complex and lack consistency. Often they are inadequate with poor integration into patient care, with the inevitable adverse impact on patient's morbidity and mortality. With this in mind, current recommendations by the American Diabetes Association (2004) and the European Diabetes Policy Group (1999) acknowledge the individual and collective impact of multiple risk factors to the wellbeing of persons with T2DM (Tables 20 and 21). Therefore, the intensive management of T2DM requires effective management of these putative risk factors. In addition to achieving glycemic control, the predominantly cardiovascular risk factors, including blood pressure and dyslipidemia, demand attention. Furthermore, there is the need for psycho-social support for persons with T2DM to achieve the defined targets (in Tables 20 and 21), which may need to be individualized.

The intention of this book is limited to exploring the role of basal insulin in the quest to achieve effective glycemic control in T2DM, acknowledging the added benefits of insulin on other components of the metabolic syndrome, and having a beneficial effect on vascular function, insulin sensitivity and various lipid parameters. The overwhelming concern is to reduce the cardiovascular burden of T2DM, given that the vast majority of persons with T2DM remain at risk, falling short of the treatment goals.

Glycemic control	
HbA$_{1c}$	<7.0%*
Preprandial plasma glucose	90–130 mg/dL (5.0–7.2 mmol/L)
Peak postprandial plasma glucose	<180 mg/dL (<10.0 mmol/L)
Blood pressure	<130/80 mmHg
Lipids	
LDL	<100 mg/dL (<2.6 mmol/L)
Triglycerides†	<150 mg.dL (<1.7 mmol/L)
HDL	>40 mg/dL (>1.1 mmol/L) ‡

* Referenced to a nondiabetic range of 4.0–6.0% using a DCCT-based assay.
† Postprandial glucose measurements should be made 1–2 h after beginning of the meal, generally peak levels in patients with diabetes.
‡ Current NCEP/ATP III guidelines suggest that in patients with triglyceride 200 mg/dL, the "non-HDL cholesterol" (total cholesterol minus HDL) be utilized. The goal is 130 mg/dL.
§ For women, it has been suggested that the HDL goal be increased by 10mg/dL.

Table 20. Summary of recommendations for adults with diabetes mellitus provided by the American Diabetes Association (ADA). The ADA recommends certain key concepts in setting glycemic goals: goals should be individualized; certain populations (children, pregnant women, and elderly) require special considerations; less intensive glycemic goals may be indicated in patients with severe or frequent hypoglycemia; more stringent glycemic goals (i.e. a normal HbA$_{1c}$ <6%) may further reduce complications at the cost of increased risk of hypoglycemia (particularly in those with T1DM); postprandial glucose may be targeted if HbA$_{1c}$ goals are not met despite reaching preprandial glucose goals. Regarding pre-and postprandial glucose values, most home use now calibrates blood glucose readings to plasma values. Plasma glucose values are 10–15% higher than whole blood glucose values, and it is crucial that people with diabetes know whether their monitor and strips provide whole blood or plasma results.

Glycemic control	Low risk	Arterial risk	Microvascular risk
HbA$_{1c}$ (%)*	≤6.5	>6.5	>7.5
Preprandial plasma glucose mg/dL (mmol/L)	<110 (6.0)	≥110 (6.0)	>125 (7.0)
Preprandial blood glucose mg/dL (mmol/L)	<100 (5.5)	≥100 (5.5)	≥110 (6.0)
Blood pressure (mmHg)	<140/85		
Lipids – mg/dL (mmol/L)			
LDL	<115 (3.0)	115-155 (3.0-4.0)	>155 (4.0)
Triglycerides	<150 (1.7)	150-200 (1.7-2.2)	>200 (2.2)
HDL	>46 (1.2)	39-46 (1.0-1.2)	<39 (1.0)

*Referenced using a DCCT-based assay.

Table 21. Summary of approach for adults with diabetes mellitus provided by the European Diabetes Policy Group (1999). The Group recommends that for each individual, targets should be set based on the risk of macrovascular (arterial) and microvascular complications. HbA$_{1c}$ should be measured every 2-6 monthly and blood lipid profile every 2-6 monthly if previously above assessment levels, otherwise annually. Blood pressure should be assessed at each consultation unless known to be below assessment levels.

Future treatment paradigms in T2DM

The treatment paradigm for T2DM has been in a state of flux and, given the clear benefits of tight glycemic control, is moving towards earlier and more effective therapeutic intervention with insulin to eliminate glucose toxicity. The introduction of basal insulin supplementation addresses the excessive hepatic glucose production, which is a key early feature in the pathophysiologic evolution of T2DM.

The application of a simple strategy of involving a "true" basal insulin supplementation for T2DM management has enormous potential of achieving the required glycemic targets, without the increased risk of hypoglycemia inherent with NPH insulin, which has hitherto been used for this purpose. Achieving and maintaining euglycemia has been an elusive goal due to the pharmacokinetic imperfections of such insulins and the resulting barrier of hypoglycemia (Cryer, 2004). The introduction of insulin glargine offers the ability to improve glycemic control, whilst concomitantly reducing the risk of hypoglycemia (Chapter 3), thereby allowing a more aggressive "treat-to-target" philosophy – the new treatment paradigm.

The application of a simple strategy involving the early introduction of basal insulin supplementation for T2DM patients inadequately controlled with existing OHAs therefore has an enormous potential. Further analysis of current treatment strategies demonstrates the unacceptable long-term glycemic burden of person with T2DM (Brown et al., 2004). The case for the use of more effective therapy, in particular the earlier introduction of insulin, is overwhelming.

The addition of a "true" basal insulin has considerable potential for the care of the person with T2DM, in particular in the context of primary care. The additional opportunity to empower the patients to self-adjust their basal insulin dose adds a further dimension.

In this chapter, we intend to provide recommendations for the introduction, dose adjustments and subsequent long-term provision of basal insulin, in the context of the overall requirements of persons with T2DM to achieve pre-defined glycemic targets. We regard achieving normal fasting blood glucose targets as an early pre-requisite in this treatment paradigm (*"fix fasting first"*), and we review the use of insulin glargine as a basal insulin supplementation in this context.

"Overcoming barriers" – the introduction of basal insulin

Where lifestyle changes have failed, the introduction of OHAs, used alone or in combination, is effective in improving glycemic control (Table 22). However, it is well recognized that they have a variable time-limited window of effectiveness, as shown in the UKPDS glucose 2 study (Wright et al., 2002) with the majority of patients afforded the benefits of insulin late in the disease process (Brown et al., 2004) with the inevitable consequences.

Regimen	Approximate reductions from baseline	
	HbA$_{1C}$ (%)	FBG (mg/dL)
Sulfonylurea + metformin	1.7	65
Sulfonylurea + pioglitazone	1.2	50
Sulfonylurea + rosiglitazone	0.9-1.4	50-60
Sulfonylurea + acarbose	1.3	40
Meglitinide + metformin	1.4	40
Pioglitazone + metformin	0.7-0.8	40-50
Rosiglitazone + metformin	0.7-0.8	50-50

Table 22. Improvements in glycemic control using different combinations of oral agents. These findings are summarized from a number of studies (DeFronzo et al., 1995; Horton et al., 1998; Coniff et al., 1995; Egan et al., 1999; Moses et al., 1999; Schneider et al., 1999; Fonseca et al., 2000).

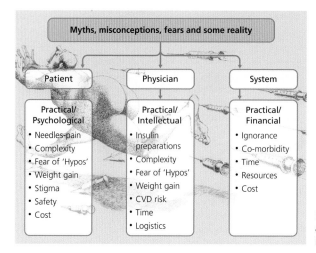

Figure 128. Patient, physician and system-related barriers to insulin therapy in T2DM.

The postponement of insulin therapy in persons with T2DM is as a result of a number of well recognized barriers (Figure 128). These **barriers** fall into a number of categories, including patient and physician concerns which are mainly about practical and psychological aspects of treatment, in addition to conceptual and societal constraints.

One of the central issues for persons with T2DM needing insulin is the requirement for subcutaneous insulin injection. This raises initial concerns about pain associated with the injection, which is easily overcome with "pen" and other delivery systems using ultra fine needles, and concerns regarding the frequency and the risk of hypoglycemia, especially at night-time. Neither can the **stigma** of having to inject be underestimated. Unfortunately for many patients, the need for insulin is perceived as a personal failure and or seen as a terminal phase of the condition. The Diabetes Attitude, Wishes and Needs (DAWN) study emphasizes the need to consider patients' attitudes and environment in addition to therapy when attempting to improve the patients' overall health status and wellbeing (discussed by Korytkowski, 2002).

The patient's concern is often compounded by the physician's resistance to initiating insulin therapy and thereby very often accepts sub-optimal glycemic control. Physicians' usual concerns include the complexity and limitations of current insulin preparations, the fear of hypoglycemia, weight gain and the misconception that the introduction of insulin can potentially increase insulin resistance and cardiovascular risk. Weight gain is usually observed in patients with glycosuria prior to improving glycemic control (UKPDS 35). The earlier introduction of more effective therapy (OHAs and or insulin) in the absence of glycosuria should not be similarly associated with weight gain. It is important to recognize that the evidence does not support insulin therapy increasing insulin resistance, or having an unfavorable influence on other known cardiovascular risk factors.

An important consideration for physicians has been the hitherto complex nature of insulin algorithms. However, this familiar concern relates largely to limitations of NPH and the insulin zinc preparations, Lente and Ultralente, which have an inadequate pharmacokinetic profile for a basal insulin (Chapter 2). Patients and physicians are concerned about the increased risk of hypoglycemia with these preparations and or their relatively poor reproducibility (due to the need for resuspension), which limits the opportunity to reach the required glycemic targets. In this context, the fact that physicians and carers are under increasing time and logistical constraints supports the need for simple, effective intervention.

It is important to recognize that the cost of insulin therapy remains a small part of the overall cost of diabetes care, especially as its early introduction aims at improving glycemic control with a consequent benefit of preventing and or limiting the progress of costly complications of diabetes.

"Overcoming complexity" – the introduction of basal insulin

A key limiting step in achieving the necessary glycemic target in the population of T2DM is the early introduction of insulin therapy. The "treat-to-target" study has clearly demonstrated the ability to achieve target glycemic control (HbA_{1c} <7%) with both NPH insulin and insulin glargine according to a predefined dose titration algorithm. However, the risk-to-benefit ratio was greater with NPH insulin due to the higher frequency of nocturnal hypoglycemia with NPH insulin at equivalent levels of glycemia, which was more in evidence at near-normoglycemia. The principal randomized clinical trials demonstrated a much reduced frequency of severe symptomatic and nocturnal hypoglycemia with insulin glargine in comparison to NPH insulin (Chapter 3). Therefore, the preferred basal insulin is insulin glargine.

BASAL INSULIN SUPPLEMENTATION – THE "TREAT-TO-TARGET" PARADIGM

The "treat-to-target" approach to attain an HbA_{1c} <7% is based on an evening injection of basal insulin glargine, whilst maintaining the current oral hypoglycemic agent(s) (Riddle, Rosenstock and Gerich, 2003). The process comprises a structured dosing algorithm to achieve fasting blood glucose levels of ≤100 mg/dL (5.5 mmol/L). This is a regimen by which basal insulin therapy can be introduced to those persons with T2DM and titrated to achieve and maintain good glycemic control in a simple fashion whilst minimizing the risk of hypoglycemia. The use of a basal insulin injection to supplement ongoing treatment with OHAs offers a simple and practical approach to overcome the complexities of introducing insulin therapy (Table 23).

In combination therapy, lower total doses of insulin are required due to the synergistic or complementary effects from the oral agents - it is suggested that each oral therapy contributes the equivalent of 10 – 20 units of insulin. Only one daily injection of insulin glargine is required, which can be given either in the morning or the evening. Unlike NPH insulin, either alone or as part of a premixed preparation, there is no need for resuspension. Doses of insulin glargine can be titrated to achieve glycemic targets in a slow, safe and simple fashion according to the original "treat-to-target" algorithm (Riddle, Rosenstock and Gerich, 2003)(Table 24). This algorithm is based on adjusting the insulin dose by 2, 4, 6,

Advantages of basal insulin therapy
Basal insulin supplementation is a physiological therapeutic option
This treatment requires a simple single injection
Basal insulin treatment effectively lowers fasting hyperglycemia
Basal insulin rarely causes severe hypoglycemia
Preliminary evidence suggests that insulin probably reduces the risk of CVD

Table 23. Advantages of basal insulin therapy in T2DM.

Forced weekly titration algorithm	
Start 10 U/day at bedtime	
Mean FPG* (mg/dL)	Insulin dose** (U/day)
100–120	2
120–140	4
140–180	6
>180	8

* use means of preceding 2 days FBG values
** increase weekly only if no severe hypoglycemia and/or no PG values <72 mg/dL (4.0 mmol/L)

Table 24. Forced weekly titration algorithm employed in "treat-to-target" study.

or 8 units per day on a weekly basis. The dose is based on the preceding two days FBG values and in the absence of any episodes of severe hypoglycemia and or PG values below 72 mg/dL (4.0 mmol/L) is increased.

Utilizing this regimen, 60% of patients reached target HbA$_{1c}$ below 7% and the mean fasting glucose was reduced to 117 mg/dL (6.5 mmol/L), with an average dose requirement for insulin glargine of 47 units per day. This original "treat-to-target" study resulted in high patient compliance, exceeding 90% and suggesting that a structured treatment algorithm is not only effective, but also simple to understand and implement by both patient-physician and patient-nurse partnerships. This original dose titration has been satisfactorily applied to other studies (Chapter 3) and has been widely adopted in clinical practice.

More recently, the algorithm was compared to a self-titration algorithm (AT.LANTUS study, Davies et al., 2004) requiring adjustment of the insulin glargine dose by 2 units every three days based on the mean fasting glucose values, whilst adopting the same targets and constraints as the "treat-to-target" algorithm. Interestingly, the self titration algorithm achieved a greater reduction in FBG compared to the original scheme that was reliant on weekly clinic contact. This was achieved with a higher insulin dose in the self-titration algorithm (35 – 46 units) compared to the original algorithm (30 - 32 units) in those patients receiving one or more OHAs, respectively (Lavalle-Gonzalez et al., 2004). There was no difference in weight gain between the two schemes.

Another study utilized the same patient self-adjustment algorithm of insulin dose (Algorithm 2 in the AT.LANTUS study) in poorly controlled persons with T2DM on 2 g metformin daily comparing bedtime insulin glargine and NPH insulin (Yki-Jarvinen et al., 2004). An additional feature of this "LANMET" study was the transfer of the home glucose values by modem to the supervising diabetes center, taking advantage of today's new communication tools. The patient sends twice-weekly fasting glucose values, but does not require a computer or any computer skills to

Mean FBG for the previous 3 consecutive days	Increase in daily basal insulin glargine dose (Units)*	
	Algorithm 1: titration at every visit	Algorithm 2: titration every 3 days
100 mg/dL and <120 mg/dL (≥5.5 mmol/L and <6.7 mmol/L)	0–2**	0–2**
120 mg/dL and <140 mg/dL (≥6.7 mmol/L and <7.8 mmol/L)	2	2
140 mg/dL and <180 mg/dL (≥7.8 mmol/L and <10 mmol/L)	4	2
≥180 mg/dL (≥10 mmol/L)	6–8**	2**

* Treat-to-target fasting blood glucose (FBG) ≤100 mg/dL (5.5 mmol/L). Titration occurred only in the absence of blood glucose levels <72 mg/dL (<4.0 mmol/L) **Magnitude of daily basal dose was at the discretion of the investigator.

Table 25. Comparison of the original "treat-to-target" weekly dose titration algorithm (Algorithm 1) and the simpler, patient-empowered titration (Algorithm 2) compared in the AT.LANTUS study.

achieve this transfer. Insulin glargine achieved a final FPG of 103 mg/dL (5.7 mmol/L) and a mean HbA_{1c} of 7.1% at a mean dose of 68 units per day, with a low incidence of symptomatic hypoglycemia, and with a 2.3 kg increase in weight. The mean HbA_{1c} reduction was marked, with an absolute reduction of 2.4% (mean values at study entry of 9.5 ± 0.1% reduced to 7.1 ± 0.1%), the largest reduction in any study using the "treat-to-target" approach and highlighting the value of this study in validating the algorithm approach to restoring effective glycemic control.

These results of the AT.LANTUS and LAN-MET studies confirm the ability of patients to self-adjust the insulin dose based on the simplest algorithm. Most notably, patients can be actively encouraged to participate fully in their own diabetes management and be empowered to make ongoing adjustments. Eventually, if target HbA_{1c} levels are not achieved after basal insulin is effectively titrated, patients will benefit by adding pre-meal insulin to control postprandial glycemic peaks.

SWITCHING TO INSULIN GLARGINE FROM OTHER INSULIN PREPARATIONS

The efficacy, safety, and ease of the "treat-to-target" strategy should be attractive to physicians, especially primary care physicians who tend to have limited time and resources compared to the hospital or speciality clinic environment. The clinical evidence presented in Chapter 3 provides evidence that this treatment paradigm should help to alleviate some of the key patient concerns about insulin therapy, overcoming doubts that insulin therapy has to be complex and poses a high risk of hypoglycemia.

If patients are inadequately controlled on NPH insulin on a once-a-day basis at bedtime and or experience unacceptable nocturnal hypoglycemic episodes, substitution to insulin glargine should be considered. It is suggested that the initial insulin glargine dose should be the same as the NPH insulin dose. Thereafter, adopt a "treat-to-target" regimen (Table 26).

Where patients are treated with NPH insulin on a twice-a-day basis with sub-optimal glycemic control and or unpredictable hypoglycemic episodes during the day or nighttime, insulin glargine should be considered. It is recommended that the starting dose should be 20% lower than the total daily dose of twice daily NPH. Thereafter, adopt a "treat-to-target" algorithm paying particular attention to fasting glucose levels whilst avoiding hypoglycemia (Table 26).

Converting patients from twice-daily premixed insulins requires a 20% lower dose than the total daily dose of the admixed insulins. The "treat-to-target" algorithm should then be adopted with respect to achieving fasting normoglycemia. Some patients may be satisfactorily controlled with the reintroduction of an

Current insulin	Insulin glargine recommendations
NPH once-daily	Convert to insulin glargine at same total daily insulin dose and titrate according to "treat-to-target" algorithm.
NPH twice-daily	Convert to insulin glargine **at a 20% reduced total daily insulin dose**; titrate according to "treat-to-target" algorithm. Additionally, patient will probably require short acting insulin agents, once FBG is corrected <100 mg/dL and the HbA_{1c} remains above 7%.
Premixed insulins	Convert to insulin glargine **at a 20% reduced total daily insulin dose**; titrate according to "treat-to-target" algorithm. Patient **will probably require supplemental insulin** (short acting insulin agents to incorporate in a progressive basal/bolus regimen).

Table 26. Recommendations on switching to insulin glargine from other insulin regimens using a "treat-to-target" algorithm

insulin secretagog pre-prandially with or without metformin; most others will require the addition of short-acting insulin to accommodate the meal insulin requirements. The meal-related insulin could be regular insulin, or a rapid-acting insulin analog such as insulin lispro, insulin aspart, or insulin glulisine (Table 26). Traditionally, supplying insulin with a twice-daily, split-mixed insulin regimen has been considered when it becomes necessary to intensify the once-daily basal insulin in combination with OHAs. However, we note that the use of premixed insulin preparations, such as 70/30 or 75/25, do not provide enough flexibility for the patient and are seldom effective to reach glycemic targets.

EDITORS COMMENTARY

Accepting the need for the early introduction of basal insulin in patients with T2DM who are poorly controlled on OHAs, the "treat-to-target" paradigm offers the basis for a simple, standardized method for the timely initiation of basal insulin in clinical practice, governed by specific targets using safe and effective dose titration algorithms (Table 27). Experience has been gained utilizing two basic algorithms – the original physician-based forced titration algorithm with an aggressive dose escalation of 2 – 8 units weekly and the alternative regimen, which is based on self-titration of 2 units of insulin per 3–7 days. There is therefore the option of adopting either of these algorithms according to the clinical circumstances.

With the increased awareness of the need for the early introduction of insulin therapy in T2DM and the proven benefit of basal insulin in achieving targets, with a low risk of hypoglycemia using insulin glargine, the evolution of dose-adjustment treatment algorithms, especially those applicable to self-management, makes the "treat-to-target" paradigm a reality to a wider patient population.

Starting basal insulin
Maintain OHA(s) at same dose (eventually reduce)
Begin single evening insulin dose (start dose of 10 U)
Adjust dose by self-monitoring fasting blood glucose
Increase the insulin dose according to chosen algorithm
Treat-to-target <100 mg/dL (5.5 mmol/L)
Modulate insulin dose if FBG <72 mg/dL (4.0 mmol/L) or if hypoglycemia

Table 27. Guidelines for starting basal insulin in patients with T2DM

References

1. Brown JB, Nichols GA, Perry A. The burden of treatment failure in type 2 diabetes. *Diabetes Care* 27:1535–1540, 2004

2. Coniff RF, Shapiro JA, Robbins D, Kleinfield R, Seaton TB, Beisswenger P, McGill JB. Reduction of glycosylated hemoglobin and postprandial hyperglycemia by acarbose in patients with NIDDM. A placebo-controlled dose-comparison study. *Diabetes Care* 1995;18:817–824.

3. Cryer PE. Diverse causes of hypoglycemia-associated autonomic failure in diabetes. *N Engl J Med* 2004;350:2272–2279.

4. Davies M, Storms F, Shutler S, Bianchi-Biscay M, Gomis R, AT.LANTUS Study Group. AT.LANTUS trial investigating treatment algorithms for insulin glargine (LANTUS®). Results of the type 2 study. *Diabetes* 2004; 53(Suppl 2):Abstract 1980 PO.

5. DeFronzo RA, Goodman AM. Efficacy of metformin in patients with non-insulin-dependent diabetes mellitus. The Multicenter Metformin Study Group. *N Engl J Med* 1995; 333:541–549.

6. Egan J, Rubin C, Mathisen A. Combination therapy with pioglitazone and metformin in patients with type 2 diabetes. *Diabetes* 1999; 48(Suppl 1):A117 Abstract 0504.

7. European Diabetes Policy Group. A desktop guide to Type 2 diabetes mellitus. *Diabet Med* 1999; 16:716–730.

8. Fonseca V, Rosenstock J, Patwardhan R, Salzman A. Effect of metformin and rosiglitazone combination therapy in patients with type 2 diabetes mellitus. *JAMA* 2000; 283:1695–1702.

9. Horton ES, Whitehouse F, Ghazzi MN, Venable TC, Whitcomb RW. Troglitazone in combination with sulfonylurea restores glycemic control in patients with type 2 diabetes. The Troglitazone Study Group. *Diabetes Care* 1998; 21:1462–1469.

10. Korytkowski M When oral agents fail: practical barriers to starting insulin. *Int J Obes Relat Metab Disord* 2002; 26(Suppl 3):S18-24.

11. Lavalle-González F, Storms F, Shutler S, Bianchi-Biscay M, Gomis R, Davies M, AT.LANTUS Study Group. Effect of basal insulin glargine therapy in type 2 patients inadequately controlled on oral antidiabetic agents: AT.LANTUS trial results. *Diabetes* 2004; 53 (Suppl 2):Abstract 12-LB.

12. Moses R, Slobodniuk R, Boyages S, Colagiuri S, Kidson W, Carter J, Donnelly T, Moffitt P, Hopkins H. Effect of repaglinide addition to metformin monotherapy on glycemic control in patients with type 2 diabetes. *Diabetes Care* 1999; 22:119–124.

13. Riddle MC, Rosenstock J, Gerich J; Insulin Glargine 4002 Study Investigators. The treat-to-target trial: randomized addition of glargine or human NPH insulin to oral therapy of type 2 diabetic patients. *Diabetes Care* 2003; 26:3080–3086.

14. Schneider R, Egan J, Houser V. Combination therapy with pioglitazone and sulfonylurea in patients with type 2 diabetes. *Diabetes* 1999; 48(Suppl 1):A106 Abstract 0458.

15. The National Cholesterol Education Program (NCEP) Expert Panel on Detection, Evaluation and Treatment of High Blood Cholesterol in Adults (Adult Treatment Panel III): Executive summary of the third report of the National Cholesterol Education Program (NCEP) Expert Panel on Detection, Evaluation and Treatment of High Blood Cholesterol in Adults (Adult Treatment Panel III). *JAMA* 2001; 285:2486–2497,

16. Wright A, Burden AC, Paisey RB, Cull CA, Holman RR; U.K. Prospective Diabetes Study Group. Sulfonylurea inadequacy: efficacy of addition of insulin over 6 years in patients with type 2 diabetes in the U.K. Prospective Diabetes Study (UKPDS 57). *Diabetes Care* 2002; 25:330-336.

17. Yki-Järvinen H, Hänninen J, Hulme S, Kauppinen-Mäkelin R, Lahdenperä S, Lehtonen R, Levanen H, Nikkiä K, Ryysy L, Tiikkainen M, Tulokas T, Virtamo H, Vahatalo M. Treat-To-Target simply – the LANMET study. *Diabetes* 2004; 53(Suppl 2):Abstract 2181-PO.

EPILOGUE

TREATMENT STRATEGIES WITH INSULIN IN TYPE 2 DIABETES

> "It is rarely possible to define a disease precisely, but it is always possible to characterize a syndrome... A syndrome is usually first glimpsed in a complex condition, associated with secondary syndromes, from which it has to be disentangled until its essential features are clear"
>
> Himsworth HP. The syndrome of diabetes mellitus and its causes. *Lancet* 1949; i:465–472.

We have come a long way in the understanding of type 2 diabetes since that visionary statement was made.

At this point early in the 21st Century, the daunting challenge from the pandemic of diabetes is almost overwhelming. With the appearance of T2DM in children, the burden of disease will be even greater in the future, with more persons expected to experience the devastating complications of chronic hyperglycemia. Despite this seemingly gloomy outlook, a new impetus exists in the diabetes and diabetes care community. The all too frequent adverse outcome in patients due to unmonitored and uncorrected blood glucose requires a new treatment paradigm that partners physicians and patients to embrace a structured and target – driven strategy for the treatment of T2DM (Rosenstock, 2004).

MILESTONE ONE – early introduction of insulin in combination with oral hypoglycemic agents

The traditional treatment approach for patients newly diagnosed with T2DM consists of lifestyle measures with recommendations for alterations in diet, to include calorie restriction and lowering the intake of saturated fats, and for increases in the level of physical activity. Successful application brings benefits in terms of weight loss and reduced glycemia in the short term, but this approach fails in the majority of patients. By the time symptomatic hyperglycemia is present, significant β cell failure is in evidence. This was confirmed by the UKPDS, which found few patients able to achieve glycemic targets without the early addition of pharmacologic agents (UKPDS 33, 1998). An interesting alternative strategy is the use of short, intensive insulin therapy to restore glycemic control, with the seeming possibility for some patients to achieve "remission" (Ilkova et al, 1997; Park and Choi, 2003; Ryan, Imes and Wallace, 2004). This approach is conceptually attractive and may have a more subtle impact on the metabolic "imprint" of the individual, potentially improving the long-term prospect of maintaining normoglycemia. However, this remains theoretical and requires validation in long term randomized controlled studies.

Patients who remain above the glycemic target level (HbA$_{1c}$ ≤7%) should proceed immediately to oral hypoglycemic agent treatment (Riddle and Rosenstock, 2004). At this point, most persons with insulin resistance are also insulin deficient and will therefore benefit from either an insulin secretagog, such as a sulfonylurea (e.g. glimepiride or gliclazide etc) or a non-sulfonylurea, such as a meglitinide (e.g. repaglinide or nateglinide) or the biguanide, metformin. The issue of which of the above agents is started first as monotherapy is really irrelevant and has no demonstrated impact on the progression of T2DM. Monotherapy with a sulfonylurea such as glimepiride will realize valuable decreases in HbA$_{1c}$, perhaps up to 2% reductions (Langtry and Balfour, 1998) depending on factors including stage of disease, the starting dose and level of compliance. Monotherapy with metformin is equally effective (DeFronzo et al., 1995) with a lesser risk of hypoglycemia and weight gain. For some patients, this can improve glycemic control for some time and does offer an interim treatment strategy.

Other persons, however, are only able to maintain glycemic control on monotherapy for a relatively short time period, due to the relentless progression of the condition.

When the single oral hypoglycemic agent approach fails to maintain blood glucose within the defined glycemic targets, escalation of the therapeutic intervention is required without delay. This theme of escalating the level of treatment as soon as the clearly defined glycemic threshold is crossed (HbA$_{1c}$ of 7%) is an essential feature of the new "treat-to-target" approach in T2DM.

Furthermore, it is highly conceivable that patients could remain consistently with a HbA$_{1c}$ <7% if combination therapy with an insulin secretagogue and an insulin sensitizer is proactively initiated from the outset of the disease sustaining near-normoglycemia and preventing the effects of glucotoxicity on the β cell. Of course, this hypothesis will need to be confirmed by long term properly controlled studies.

Indeed, a major component of the overall glycemic burden to which patients are exposed reflects the delay in adjusting therapy to meet the increasing requirement for intervention over time (Brown, Nichols and Perry, 2004). In a recent study, the average HbA$_{1c}$ reported in patients before metformin was added to sulfonylurea treatment was unacceptably high at 9.4 % (Brown and Nichols, 2003). This study reported that the average patient accumulates 10 HbA$_{1c}$-years of glycemic burden >7% before insulin is commenced. Clearly, a change in the approach to glucose-lowering treatment is required.

Various combinations of oral agents will bring improved glycemic control due to the potential additive or synergistic action. However, despite intensive and maximal oral therapy, eventually this approach may be insufficient to maintain the necessary glycemic control due to the late stage of the condition and reflecting the inadequacies of these agents at an advanced stage of the disease. Increasing dysglycemia reflects an increasing deficiency in β cell function in the face of insulin insensitivity.

UKPDS 57 provided important data on the need for, and efficacy of, insulin in addition to sulfonylurea treatment (Wright et al., 2002). In a 6-year follow up of 826 newly diagnosed patients with T2DM, more than half of those allocated to sulfonylurea required addition of insulin, because of fasting plasma glucose levels above 108 mg/dL (6 mmol/L). Those randomized to an intensive policy of insulin and sulfonylurea maintained significantly better glycemic control compared to those patients receiving insulin alone and did not experience additional weight gain. Many studies (>30) and meta-analyses described in the 1990's (listed and reviewed in Yki-Järvinen, 2001 & DeWitt and Hirsch, 2003) consistently demonstrated that glycemic control is similar or improved with combination insulin and oral agents. There are other additive benefits, however with combination oral agents and insulin therapy that include the simplicity of a single basal insulin injection, reduced monitoring and dose sparing effects, with potentially less weight gain and less hypoglycemia. This clinical evidence supports the role of insulin in combination with oral agents, a role that has been widely accepted. The earlier introduction of insulin is recommended and early addition a priority once the glycemic target has been breached, which will secure an improved metabolic status for the person with T2DM.

MILESTONE TWO – introduction of "treat-to-target" algorithms with basal insulin

The pharmacokinetic imperfections of the previously available long-acting insulin preparations, in particular NPH insulin, have been a key component in the decision to delay insulin intervention. NPH is not ideal once-daily insulin, with a peak of activity 4-6 hours after subcutaneous injection and an inadequate duration of action (12–16 hours). The need for more complex insulin treatment algorithms to account for the poor kinetic characteristics is a major barrier to insulin initiation. However, the ultimate barrier is hypoglycemia, both the fear of, and the reality of hypoglycemia.

Hypoglycemia has a major negative impact

on the quality of life of people with diabetes that cannot be underestimated. It is the occurrence of hypoglycemia that "precludes maintenance of euglycemia during the lifetime of a person with diabetes and, thus, full realization of the well-established benefits of glycemic control" (Cryer 2004). We know well that there is an inevitable 'trade-off' between a therapeutic strategy employing the adequate dose of insulin to achieve glycemic control and that utilizing a dose least likely to cause hypoglycemia. Insulin glargine is the first long-acting recombinant insulin to provide a "true" basal insulin supplementation, when administered within a defined treatment strategy. The supplementation of oral pharmacotherapy with once daily insulin glargine to achieve and maintain target HbA_{1c} ≤7% with forced but structured dosing algorithms sets the new paradigm for treatment in T2DM.

Randomized trials support the clinical utility of supplementing oral pharmacotherapy with once-daily insulin glargine to achieve and maintain target HbA_{1c} levels ≤7%. The "treat-to-target" study showed that using a simple forced titration of insulin dose within a defined algorithm, one third of patients achieved target glycemic control (HbA_{1c} ≤7%) without a single episode of nocturnal hypoglycemia, in contrast to NPH insulin (one quarter fewer patients reached this endpoint)(Riddle, Rosenstock and Gerich, 2003). Overall, 60% of patients achieved target glycemic control with both insulins, but with markedly reduced hypoglycemia with insulin glargine compared to NPH insulin.

Further relatively large studies have validated this "treat-to-target" approach (detailed in Chapter 3). These studies have shown that flexible insulin dosing (morning or bedtime) does not compromise efficacy or safety outcome (Fritsche et al., 2003; Standl et al., 2003), the value of earlier insulin intervention in the disease course, resulting in reduced dose requirement, reduced hypoglycemia, and less weight gain (Fach et al., 2004) and the positive impact on glycemic control in very large numbers of patients enrolled in "real-world" clini-

cal practice studies (Schreiber et al., 2004).

A common consideration as therapy is escalated is the option of adding a third oral hypoglycemic agent as opposed to initiating insulin. Important concerns with three oral agents include the potential for an additive risk of adverse events, dose adjustments which may become complex and cost considerations. In a study comparing the efficacy, safety, and cost of managing persons who have failed on two oral agent therapy by adding either a third class of oral agent or switching treatment to insulin 70/30 mix twice-daily plus metformin, 70/30 mix plus metformin was as effective as triple oral therapy in lowering HbA_{1c} and FPG values (Schwartz et al., 2003). However, the triple oral regimen was not as cost effective, and a high percentage of subjects did not complete this regimen due to lack of efficacy or side effects. The findings of this study were also informative by showing the limitations of premixed insulin in reaching effective glycemic control. Only one third of patients reached the target of 7% on premixed insulin with high frequency of hypoglycemia, comparing poorly with the 60% achieving target in the "treat-to-target" study with lower levels of hypoglycemia (Riddle, Rosenstock and Gerich, 2003). Indeed, the "treat-to-target" study has raised the standard for the proper design and interpretation of future insulin studies in T2DM.

A number of studies comparing premixed insulin have being described recently. The LAPTOP study has shown that insulin glargine with continued oral agents is a more effective treatment strategy than the common approach of switching to premixed insulin and stopping oral therapy (Janka et al., 2004). Additional analyses of this study await full publication. Other studies have been conducted with premixed (Malone et al., 2004a; Malone et al., 2004b), but these studies did not effectively titrate the insulin glargine dose using aggressive algorithms to FPG 100 mg/dL. The titration algorithm is always most critical to interpret the results in regards to the proportion of patients reaching HbA_{1c} target and relationship with hypoglycemia and therefore the findings do not fully answer the questions physicians are interested in when comparing insulin glargine with premixed insulins.

The once-daily flexible dosing of insulin glargine, and its smooth profile of activity associated with fewer episodes of nocturnal hypoglycemia, make it a practical therapeutic intervention to transform T2DM management. The most recent step taken in elucidating this new standard of care has been defining the process of effectively and safely increasing the insulin dose. This can be undertaken safely, effectively and with patient empowerment to self adjust to normalize the fasting glucose and thus maintain the target glycemic level of 7%, as highlighted by the preliminary reports of AT.LANTUS (Davies et al., 2004) and LANMET (Yki-Järvinen et al., 2004) studies. The structured insulin dosing algorithm based on self-monitored blood glucose levels and self-adjustment of dose by 2 units every 3 days if fasting glucose is above 100 mg/dL on 3 consecutive mornings, empowers the patient to actively participate in their own management. This approach is widely translatable to general practice to allow physicians to facilitate the move from oral pharmacotherapy to early addition of basal insulin glargine if glycemic targets are not met.

The ultimate goal of lifelong maintenance of euglycemia in persons with diabetes had remained elusive because of the pharmacokinetic imperfections of insulin preparations, such as NPH insulin, and thereby the resulting barrier of hypoglycemia to the achievement of the target glycemic level. The end of this milestone is to achieve the required glycemic target with a simple and safe treatment algorithm involving insulin glargine to allow the attainment of required fasting glucose values (100 mg/dL) with reduced hypoglycemic risk. This first step of insulin replacement therapy establishes the conceptual message of "fix fasting first"

MILESTONE THREE – "basal/bolus" physiologic insulin replacement

Basal insulin provision is intended to inhibit hepatic glucose production in an attempt to normalize fasting blood glucose. When normalization is achieved, but the HbA_{1c} remains above the defined HbA_{1c} target of 7%, attention should then be focused on assessing and correcting the post-prandial glucose excursions. Recent evidence provides some insight into the relative contributions of fasting and postprandial hyperglycemia to the glycemic burden in patients treated on oral agents without insulin (Monnier, Lapinski and Colette, 2003) but validates this approach of "fix fasting first", and then escalating therapy to include prandial insulin as required when the HbA_{1c} exceeds 7%. In those patients with well controlled glycemia, it is the postprandial glucose excursions that are the predominant factor in the glycemic burden, and proper intervention with prandial insulin can further improve glycemic control when basal insulin therapy has already been maximized. The decision to introduce a prandial insulin preparation (a rapid acting analog), should be on the basis of prandial glucose monitoring. The stepwise introduction at the main meal first and then covering additional meals will be determined over time according to the need (postprandial blood glucose) and the patient's lifestyle. This basal/bolus insulin approach is the mainstay of the management of patients with T1DM, and increasingly should find a role in patients with T2DM (Rosenstock, 2001). Initially advancing with a twice daily regimen of basal insulin glargine in the morning in combination with oral agents and a second injection of a rapid-acting analog before the main meal will provide a flexible regimen for insulin adjustments based on specific targets. Patients should not be left with excess glycemic burden for extended periods and an aggressive strategy to maintain glycemic control to the target level will bring well-being to the patient and counter the dreaded long-term complications of diabetes.

Fifty five years on from Himsworth's remarkable work, the challenge has changed. The essential features of type 2 diabetes and the terrible long-term consequences of hyperglycemia are clear. Defining glycemic targets has been a critical milestone, with restoration of glycemic control offering persons with type 2 diabetes relief from their dysmetabolic malaise. The treatment approach, moving from oral hypoglycemic agents to insulin, partnered with patient glucose monitoring to define the metabolic status, allows appropriate therapy optimization through escalation, once the glycemic threshold has been crossed. It is the use of early basal insulin treatment with oral hypoglycemic agents, with special focus on normalizing fasting blood glucose, and eventually, close control of the meal-time requirement through basal/bolus replacement strategies, that provide the keys to effective management in the 21st Century.

References

1. Brown JB, Nichols GA. Slow response to loss of glycemic control in type 2 diabetes mellitus. *Am J Manag Care* 2003; 9:213-217.

2. Brown JB, Nichols GA, Perry A.The burden of treatment failure in type 2 diabetes. *Diabetes Care* 2004; 27:1535-1540.

3. Cryer PE. Diverse causes of hypoglycemia-associated autonomic failure in diabetes. *N Engl J Med* 2004; 350:2272-2279.

4. Davies M, Storms F, Shutler S, Bianchi-Biscay M, Gomis R. AT.LANTUS Study Group. AT.LANTUS trial investigating treatment algorithms for insulin glargine (LANTUS®). Results of the type 2 study. Diabetes 2004; 53(Suppl 2):Abstract 1980–PO.

5. DeFronzo RA, Goodman AM. Efficacy of metformin in patients with non-insulin-dependent diabetes mellitus. The Multicenter Metformin Study Group. *N Engl J Med* 1995; 333:541-549.

6. DeWitt DE, Hirsch IB. Outpatient insulin therapy in type 1 and type 2 diabetes mellitus: scientific review. *JAMA* 2003; 289:2254-2264.

7. Fach E-M, Busch K, Anderesi Z-K, Schweitzer M.A, Standl E, HOE901/4009 Study Group. Efficacy of insulin glargine in type 2 diabetes: effect at different stages of disease. *Diabetes* 2004; 53(Suppl 2): Abstract 524P.

8. Fritsche A, Schweitzer MA, Haring HU. Glimepiride combined with morning insulin glargine, bedtime neutral protamine hagedorn insulin, or bedtime insulin glargine in patients with type 2 diabetes. A randomized, controlled trial. *Ann Intern Med* 2003; 138:952–959.

9. Ilkova H, Glaser B, Tunckale A, Bagriacik N, Cerasi E. Induction of long-term glycemic control in newly diagnosed type 2 diabetic patients by transient intensive insulin treatment. *Diabetes Care* 1997; 20:1353-1356.

10. Janka H, Plewe G, Kliebe-Frisch C, Schweitzer M.A, Yki-Järvinen H. Starting insulin for type 2 diabetes with insulin glargine added to oral agents vs. twice-daily premixed insulin alone. *Diabetes* 2004; 53 (Suppl 2): Abstract 548-P.

11. Langtry HD, Balfour JA. Glimepiride. A review of its use in the management of type 2 diabetes mellitus. *Drugs* 1998; 55:563-584.

12. Malone J.K, Holcombe J.H, Campaigne B.N, Kerr L.F. Insulin lispro mix 75/25 compared to insulin glargine in patients with type 2 diabetes new to insulin therapy *Diabetes* 2004a; 53(Suppl 2):Abstract 576-P.

13. Malone J.K, Bai S, Campaigne B.N, Reviriego J, Augendre-Ferrante B. Targeting postprandial rather than fasting blood glucose results in better overall glycemic control in patients with type 2 diabetes. *Diabetes* 2004b; 53(Suppl 2):Abstract 577P.

14. Monnier L, Lapinski H, Colette C. Contributions of fasting and postprandial plasma glucose increments to the overall diurnal hyperglycemia of type 2 diabetic patients: variations with increasing levels of HbA_{1c}. *Diabetes Care* 2003; 26:881-885.

15. Park S, Choi SB. Induction of long-term normoglycemia without medication in Korean type 2 diabetes patients after continuous subcutaneous insulin infusion therapy. *Diabetes Metab Res Rev* 2003; 19:124-130.

16. Riddle MC, Rosenstock J, Gerich J. On behalf of the insulin glargine 4002 study investigators: the Treat-to-Target Trial. *Diabetes Care* 2003; 26:3080–2086.

17. Riddle M, Rosenstock J. Type 2 Diabetes: Oral monotherapy and combination therapy. In: The CADRE Handbook of Diabetes Management. New York: Medical Information Press, 2004.

18. Rosenstock J. Insulin Therapy: Optimizing Control in Type 1 and Type 2 Diabetes. *Clinical Cornerstone* 2001; 4:50-64.

19. Rosenstock J. Basal Insulin Supplementation in Type 2 Diabetes: Refining the Tactics. *Am J Med* 2004; 116:10S-16S.

20. Rosenstock J, Sugimoto D, Strange P, Stewart J, Soltes-Rak E, Dailey G. Triple therapy in type 2 diabetes (T2DM): Benefits of insulin glargine (GLAR) over rosiglitazone (RSG) when added to combination therapy of sulfonylurea plus Metformin (SU+MET) in insulin-naive patients *Diabetes* 2004; 53(Suppl 2): Abstract 609P.

21. Ryan EA, Imes S, Wallace C. Short-term intensive insulin therapy in newly diagnosed type 2 diabetes. *Diabetes Care* 2004; 27:1028–1032.

22. Schreiber S.A, Schneider K, Schweitzer MA. Insulin glargine in type 2 diabetes: An observational study of everyday practice. *Diabetes* 2004; 53(Suppl 2): Abstract 2043-PO.

23. Schwartz S, Sievers R, Strange P, Lyness WH, Hollander P; INS-2061 Study Team. Insulin 70/30 mix plus metformin versus triple oral therapy in the treatment of type 2 diabetes after failure of two oral drugs: efficacy, safety, and cost analysis. *Diabetes Care*. 2003 26:2238-2243.

24. Standl E, Maxeiner S, Schweitzer MA. Incidence of nocturnal hypoglycemia in patients with Type 2 diabetes is comparable when either morning or bedtime insulin glargine is co-administered with glimepiride. *Diabetologia* 2003; 46(Suppl 2):A6 Abstract 11.

25. U.K. Prospective Diabetes Study (UKPDS) Group: Intensive blood-glucose control with sulphonylureas or insulin compared with conventional treatment and risk of complications in patients with type 2 diabetes (UKPDS 33). *Lancet* 1998; 352:837–853.

26. Wright A, Burden AC, Paisey RB, Cull CA, Holman RR; U.K. Prospective Diabetes Study Group. Sulfonylurea inadequacy: efficacy of addition of insulin over 6 years in patients with type 2 diabetes in the U.K. Prospective Diabetes Study (UKPDS 57). *Diabetes Care* 2002; 25:330–336.

27. Yki-Järvinen H. Combination therapies with insulin in type 2 diabetes. *Diabetes Care*. 2001; 24:758-767.

28. Yki-Järvinen H, Hänninen J, Hulme S, Kauppinen-Mäkelin R, Lahdenperä S, Lehtonen R, Levanen H, Nikkiä K, Ryysy L, Tiikkainen M, Tulokas T, Virtamo H, Vahatalo M. Treat To Target simply – the LANMET study. *Diabetes* 2004; 53(Suppl 2):Abstract 2181-PO.